MEDICAL ETHICS AN INTRODUCTION

To
Jennifer

Kenneth Kearon

Medical Ethics: An Introduction

THE COLUMBA PRESS • APCK

First published in 1995 by
THE COLUMBA PRESS
93 The Rise, Mount Merrion, Blackrock, Co Dublin, Ireland
and
APCK
St Ann's Bookcentre, Dawson Street, Dublin 2

Cover by Bill Bolger
Origination by The Columba Press
Printed in Ireland by
Colour Books Ltd, Dublin

ISBN 1 85607 125 1

B 90 943 /171·7
£6 ·99

Table of Contents

Introduction

From being a cinderella subject a few years ago, medical ethics has leapt to centre stage of public discussion and debate. Traditional areas of debate like abortion and euthanasia have been joined by controversies about assisted conception and clinical research. Less sensational subjects such as privacy and confidentiality are increasingly important in day to day medical practice.

The purpose of this book is to provide a readily accessible introduction to this field for those involved in or concerned with ethics in medical practice. They include doctors, nurses, paramedics, health administrators, clergy, and the general public, who more and more are being drawn into the debates. My intention is simply to introduce readers to some of the ethical aspects of a number of areas of medicine, to help them recognise the issues and find their way around the debates, and then to make up their own mind on the subject. The discussion of a number of issues has been left open-ended deliberately.

An inductive method has been used – getting in quickly to the discussion of specific questions and concerns and allowing principles to emerge, which can then be applied to newer areas of debate. As part of this process, significant statements in the text are printed in italics. The basis is Christian, but I hope that sufficient common ground will be established to enable a discussion with those of other faiths and of none. The aim is to explore together, rather than to teach.

Writing today always runs up against the limitation of the English language with respect to the pronouns 'he' and 'she'. For convenience I have referred to a patient as 'he', and to a doc-

tor as 'she'. Also, for brevity, I have referred to any member of
the medical profession as a doctor, though usually the designa-
tion could equally refer to a nurse, or other health worker.

CHAPTER 1

The Right to Life

Human rights and the right to life

We cannot proceed very far on the subject of ethics without discussing the issue of human rights because such rights are at the heart of all ethical thinking.

Rights have been defined as 'Powers or privileges to which an individual has a just claim such that he or she can demand that they be not infringed or suspended'.[1] The claim mentioned in this definition is the claim that one individual has on another person. The rights we enjoy are dependent on the willingness of others to allow them. So while basic rights are individual in nature, they depend on a community to respect them.

The most basic right of all is the 'right to life', often regarded as the right from which all others are derived. It can be argued that without that right no other right makes sense, and that it is by teasing out the implications of the right to life that we find the basis of all other rights.

The right to life is the right to enjoy the life we have, the right not to have our life arbitrarily ended or put at serious risk by others. It leads on to secondary rights to determine, within limits, the way we choose to live that life, to the rights to autonomy and privacy and so on, and from there to the right to the means to enable those rights, such as education, health care and to work. It is because these and many other rights are derived from the right to life, that it is described as a *basic* right.

Here we must make a distinction in terminology. We have described the right to life as *basic*, because without it most other human rights do not make sense. But that does not mean that the right to life is *absolute*. To say a right is absolute implies that there can never be any exceptions to it under any circumstances. There are very few situations where the right to life can legimately be taken away from a person, but such do exist and must be recognised.

Such exceptions centre on the rights of others to *their* right to life. We have already seen that rights only exist in community, and we can only assume rights for ourselves with consequent demands on others to provide for those rights (*cf* the definition of rights above) if we acknowledge the rights of others and accept *their* demands on us to ensure *their* rights. This applies to the right to life as to any other right. We can only claim the right to life for ourselves if we are prepared to grant that right to life to others.

This is at the heart of the exceptions to the right to life. By threatening the right to life of others we loose our own right. The most obvious example of this is self-defence. If A threatens the life of B, and the only way B can defend his/her life is to kill A, then B's action can be justified on the grounds of self-defence and he won't be guilty of murder, provided no other option was open to B.

A different version of this occurs when civil authorities empower certain groups, usually the police or armed forces, to protect the lives of its citizens. If someone seriously threatens the life of another (e.g. in attempted murder, kidnapping or armed robbery) then a policeman will not be culpable if he kills the criminal in order to protect others, again provided there was no other way of achieving this protection.

This has been a long route to make a simple but very important point – that *while the right to life is a basic right, in that it is the basis for all other human rights, it is not an absolute right, because in certain very exceptional cases one may legitimately take the life of another.*

Sources of the right to life

Where does the right to life come from? It is a virtually universal right, found in every society, and it has a number of sources.

Historically, in Western societies anyway, the right comes from religious belief. One of the central tenets of Christianity is that God created the world in which we live, and gave life to human-kind. Because life is God-given no one has the right to take human life, not even one's own. Human life is sacred.

However this does not mean that only religious people believe in the right to life. It is possible to defend that right on purely secular grounds. Such arguments usually take either of two forms:

(a) The right to life is a natural right – something inherent in our humanity. There is a natural drive to preserve our own exist-ence, and the recognition of this drive towards preservation in others is the basis of the right to life.

(b) Alternatively, we can argue that there is an assumed contract or agreement among the members of every society that certain basic needs will be guaranteed in order for that society to func-tion. One of these is the right to life which is presupposed in any dealings we have with other people. To give a very simple ex-ample: you would not enter a shop or do business with another person, if there was a strong likelihood he or she might kill you!

What does 'life' mean?

Talk of the right to life assumes we have a clear understanding of what 'life' is, but this is far from certain. Much ethical debate centres on the definition of the boundaries of life (when does life begin? when does it end?), but the question of what life itself is is a different question.

To start with a very basic question – if we walked into a room and saw a person lying on the floor, how would we know that person is alive rather than dead? Quite a number of criteria would be appropriate – if the person moved or spoke, or eyelids fluttered, or we could see him breathing. If all these proved neg-ative we would be pushed towards more 'medical' criteria like body warmth or pulse. We shall return to the medical criteria in another chapter, but its important to note the sorts of character-istics we look for in ordinary usage to describe being alive; we look for movement, speech or reaction to any form of stimulus.

It is reasonable, I believe, to say that for most people, being alive means being able to relate in some way – either by relating to other people by speech or other human contact, to oneself by self-awareness or memory, or by relating to one's environment by movement, sensation or reaction to external stimuli. This is our 'ordinary language' understanding of what it is to be alive, and the more 'medical' definitions are relevant because they provide the necessary prerequisites for such life. However mere breathing and circulation in the absence of anything else, while sufficient for saying someone is not dead, is not equivalent to saying someone is alive – we might prefer to describe it as 'mere existence' or 'a vegetable existence'.

As Richard McCormick has pointed out, 'life' can have two meanings: '(1) a state of human functioning (or capacity there-of), of well-being; or (2) the existence of vital and metabolic processes with no human functioning or capacity'.[2] It is the for-mer sense of 'life' we mean when we talk of the sanctity of human life or its value; it is that life we are concerned to pre-serve and enhance. The second view is associated with medical vitalism – the concern and attribution of value to the functioning of the human organism in itself. Few people are vitalists, but the confusion of the two meanings can cause difficulties in medical ethics.

Points for discussion or reflection

1. Upholding human rights in society usually involves balancing one person's rights against another's. What special difficulties arise when trying to balance one person's right to life against another's?

2. War propaganda often involves dehumanising the enemy in an attempt to justify denying him the right to life. Discuss some twentieth-century examples of this.

3. Discuss the 'ordinary language' definition of life with refer-ence to severe mental or physical handicap.

Notes:

1. J.F. Childress and J. Macquarrie (eds), *A New Dictionary of Christian Ethics*, (SCM,1986), p 556.
2. R. McCormick, *How Brave a New World?* (London, 1981) p 396.

CHAPTER 2

The Person as Subject

Most contacts between patients and the medical profession are not matters of life and death – most would be described as part of routine medical care. The great moral questions about the boundaries of life are not raised, yet there is a number of ethical issues surrounding all contacts between patient and doctor, and it is to some of these that we now turn.

How do we ensure the integrity of the person in such contacts? How is the patient's dignity to be respected? The key features of personhood remain – the ability or capacity to relate and to be the subject of human functioning (i.e. to be the one who functions). The fact that one is a subject means that one can make decisions and ought to be allowed to do so; that each person has a conscience which ought to be respected, and that consent must be sought and obtained before any treatment proceeds, and so on.

There are certain assumptions made by a patient when he enters a doctor's surgery or a hospital, all of them expressing his dignity as a person. The overriding assumption is that the doctor will act only in the best interests of the patient, to the best of her ability; further that there will be truthfulness in all their dealings one with another; and also that strict confidentiality will be observed. All of these mark out the basis of the patient/doctor relationship. In this area, the most basic concept is 'autonomy'.

Autonomy

The best known definition of 'autonomy' comes from Immanuel Kant, the eighteenth century German philosopher, who said that all rational beings have the capacity to act in a consistent moral manner. The implicit corollary is that they should be allowed to do so.

What Kant is saying is that every person has the ability to understand notions of right and wrong and to act accordingly. It does
not of course mean that everyone will agree on what is right, nor
that once understood each person will always do what is right.
This belief is central to 'respect for the person' – a phrase often
used to indicate and safeguard the right of every person to make
his or her own decisions and to have those decisions respected
by others.

This freedom however does not imply that one can choose to do
whatever one wants and to have that decision respected by others.
The major limitation on this freedom is that one must be prepared to allow the same degree of freedom to everyone else. I
cannot use my freedom in such a way that it restricts the freedom of others. For example, my freedom to do what I like in my
own home will be restricted if I use that freedom (say by storing
explosives or playing very loud music) in a way which impairs
the rights and freedoms of others to live in safety, or to enjoy a
reasonable degree of peace and quiet. My freedom to do what I
like with my car is restricted by the right of others to travel without unnecessary risk. Much law is concerned with balancing the
rights of one individual against others, and with setting limits
on human freedom.

The possession of this freedom to determine one's own life, to
make decisions, and to control what is done to oneself is what
we call *autonomy*, and it should be obvious that the concept is
central to medical ethics. The whole thrust of medicine centres
on the health and well-being of the patient as person, and this
begins with recognising that *the patient is the primary decision-
maker with respect to his own health and medical care.*

Conscience

A person making moral judgements is, we say, exercising
his/her conscience. Conscience has been defined as 'the whole
person passing moral judgements on issues of right and
wrong'.[1] It is not just our reason nor is it just our emotions, it is
all that we are that is the agent of conscience.

A central feature of conscience is its ability to give reasons for its decisions and it is this that distinguishes it from emotions or gut reactions. This is important. It is not uncommon for individuals to declare something as morally wrong when what they really mean is that they find it personally distasteful.

One sometimes meets this, for example, in discussions about the use of live animals in research. Moral arguments can be made both for and against such research, and it is on the basis of such arguments that one should make a moral decision on the issue (i.e. by the exercise of conscience). However many people decide their attitude solely on an emotional basis – they find the idea of animal experiments repulsive and sickening, and are opposed to them for that reason. Of course each person is free to decide the issue for him/herself on any chosen basis, but it is incorrect to describe the latter decision as conscience or the experiments as morally wrong on those grounds.

Consent

Consent is when two or more people agree in conscience on something, be it marriage or a medical procedure. The features of consent are freedom (i.e. one must have some degree of choice to do or not do what is proposed) and the possession of appropriate information on which to base the decision by each person involved. To take the marriage example – it would not be a genuine marriage if one person made the vows literally at gunpoint, nor would it be a marriage if one or other partner did not understand what marriage was.

Consent in medicine: Consent is basic to all medical procedures and treatments. Both the doctor and the patient must consent before a particular course can be followed. Each patient's autonomy must be respected – each has a right to decide whether or not to accept any treatment or to refuse to continue with treatment, and has the right to have that decision respected even if it is not in his best interest to do so. No doctor can force treatment on any patient.

The doctor must also consent. The fact that a patient demands a form of treatment does not thereby oblige a doctor to provide it. *Both* must agree, and the doctor may withold her consent and so refuse to treat a patient.

In consenting, both doctor and patient are agreeing in conscience on a way to proceed. For each person that decision must be based on appropriate information. It is obvious that a doctor will be conversant with the procedure and usually will have been the person who suggested it. Her decision will be fully informed.

It cannot be assumed that the patient will understand the proposed treatment, yet for him to consent he too must have sufficient information and know what his options are. Normally the responsibility for providing that information falls on the doctor concerned. This confers considerable power and responsibility on her. She controls the information the patient has, and it can be a temptation to provide only that information which will lead the patient to decide in the way she recommends.

For example, a patient is diagnosed as having a condition which can be treated either by an operation or by drug therapy. Either treatment is possible, but the doctor believes that with this patient an operation is preferable and has the best chance of success. In informing the patient (who presumably has no knowledge of medicine) it would be possible to tell him that surgery is the only treatment available, or to present the option of drug therapy in such a way as to make it sound less of an option than in fact it is, so causing him to agree to surgery. The doctor may justify this by saying that it is in the patient's best interest, but in fact she has denied or limited that patient's important right to choose what is done to him and so has diminished his autonomy – the patient cannot genuinely be said to have consented.

Conversely, if the doctor does explain the options clearly and gives her considered opinion that surgery is the best way forward, and the patient still chooses drug therapy, the doctor is not obliged to treat the patient in that way and may refuse and refer the patient to another doctor. Both doctor and patient must freely decide on the way to proceed, and neither should be pressured by the other, nor by anyone else for that matter.

Expressing consent: The most obvious way of expressing consent is by saying or implying 'yes'. This is what happens in a GP's surgery when a patient accepts a prescription, or in a casualty department when a doctor says 'I'll have to give you an injection', and the patient does not object. In such cases the patient is obviously in control of himself, understands the treatment, which is generally uncontroversial anyway, and can opt out of treatment at any time. However, not all circumstances are as straightforward as this.

Some examples of consent: (1) The consent form: With a general anaesthetic there will be a period when the patient will not be able to exercise control or opt out. This means that another method has to be found whereby a patient can consent and thus remain in control. The usual way is by means of a 'consent form'. Here the doctor states in writing what it is proposed to do while the patient is unconscious, and if the patient understands and agrees to this he can give his consent in writing, usually by signing the form, so that there can be no misunderstanding as to the nature and extent of the consent. The key moral issue is that the patient fully understands what he is consenting to and does so without pressure. Often such consent is very general, since the available options will not be known until the operation has begun, and it is sensible to proceed with treatment at that point, rather than wait for further consent and another operation. While such general consent (sometimes expressed by the instruction 'and proceed' on the consent form) may make sense, it is very important that the patient understands the extent of the wide powers he is giving the doctor in such a case.

(2) Assumed consent: If a patient is brought into a casualty department unconscious and unaccompanied it is reasonable to assume that the patient would consent for such treatment as is necessary either to save his life or return him to consciousness or to deal with other urgent medical conditions. However any further treatment which is non-essential ought to be delayed until consent is obtained.

(3) Next-of-kin consent: It is widely accepted that when a person is unable to express consent the consent of his next-of-kin may be sought and accepted as consent on his behalf. This is morally acceptable in most cases because it can be generally assumed that

the next-of-kin will know the patient best and so will act in the best interest of the patient and will have his well-being at heart. However, if there is any suspicion that this is not the case, and that the next-of-kin may have other motives, or if the action of consenting or witholding consent is not obviously being exercised to the patient's benefit, then the doctor is entitled to query that consent and the relative's right to express it.

(4) Parents and their children: Children and minors usually do not have the right to consent to treatment on their own behalf; parents or guardians act on their behalf. However, as with next-of-kin consent, this consent is limited to consent to what is in the best interests of the child. Parents do not have the right to endanger the lives or health of their children unnecessarily.[2]

This principle is behind the reports of court cases in which parents who have refused to consent to a blood transfusion for their child are taken to court by the hospital. The refusal is often for sincere religious reasons. In such cases the court usually decides that while adults have the right to refuse blood transfusions for themselves and perhaps endanger their lives in so doing, they do not have a similar right on behalf of their children if it is not in the interest of their physical well-being. In such cases the court (acting on behalf of society) exercises consent on behalf of the child.

Privacy and confidentiality

Implicit in the control of one's life expressed in the concept of autonomy is the right to control what information others may have about oneself. To have information about someone else is a form of power and, depending on its content, can be used to exercise a form of control over another person. It follows then that for a person to be genuinely free and autonomous they must have control over the information others have about them.

One aspect of this is the introduction of Data Protection Acts in many countries. This is a response to the recent ability, with computers and other forms of information storage and transmission, for information gained in one context to be made available very easily to others in another context. The principle behind such acts is that in general (though with some limitations and exceptions) no one may have information about someone which the person himself is unaware of, and that someone in possession of information must not pass it on to another without permission. For example, most would agree that it would be wrong for your doctor to know you were HIV positive without telling you, and wrong for your bank manager to pass information about your bank account on to, say, an advertising agency without your permission.

Data Protection Acts give you the right of access to information about you that someone may hold, and also prevent the sharing or selling of that information to another person or body without your consent. Limitations and exceptions do exist. They are usually based on what is genuinely in your best interest, or in order to protect society. The holding and sharing of information by police forces is a good example of the latter.

All of this is an expression of the basic principle that *you have the right to control access to personal information and that a person with such information must act responsibly and in accordance with your wishes.*

It should be obvious that such principles are basic to medical practice also. In order for a doctor to treat you properly she must have access to a lot of personal information which most people would not disclose to the general public – information about age, weight, personal and family history, lifestyle, sometimes even one's financial circumstances, and so on.

Access to such personal information is very necessary in medicine but it confers on the person to whom it is given serious responsibilities. What is happening is that the patient is extending his privacy to include the doctor, and so the doctor is bound by the patient's own privacy. The doctor therefore has no right to share information gained in such situations with anyone else without the patient's permission.

However since the information is given in a medical context for a medical purpose it is generally assumed that relevant information may be shared with other health professionals concerned with the patient. Thus, information given to a GP may be shared with a consultant, physiotherapist or similar person to whom the patient is referred, and information supplied on admission to a hospital can be recorded on a file to which members of the medical team have access, but it does not mean that anyone who is a health professional may have information about any patient in the hospital (e.g. a relative or friend who happens to work in the same hospital). The same strict confidentiality applies to personal non-medical information which a patient may choose to tell a doctor, or more commonly, a nurse.

A patient's right to know

The doctor's relationship is with the patient and it is to him that the doctor is answerable. It follows, therefore, that it is the patient who should be told any relevant information about his condition and treatment. Much of what has already been said about privacy is also relevant in this context since details about one's health are personal and so a doctor would want very good reasons for not telling a patient the full details about his condition. Yet this isn't always the practice in fact. Most people will know of at least one case where a patient was not told the full extent of his illness, even though family and friends have known, and may even have shared in the deception.

Sometimes such a situation may arise because the doctor has not had the courage to face the patient directly with bad news. More often, the news has been told to a near relative first, and the relative has said that the patient must not be told, and the doctor has acquieced. Occasionally, from her knowledge of the patient, the doctor has decided that it is not in the best interest of the patient to know the truth about a terminal illness. All such situations may be further complicated if the patient realises he is not being told the full truth and begins to ask awkward questions.

This all too common scenario is best approached from an ethical perspective by starting with basics. First, we have already said that the doctor's relationship is with her patient, and that patient has a right to know all relevant information about his health – it is part of one's right to information about oneself which others may possess. Not to tell the patient significant information is to betray his trust. For a doctor to tell the patient wrong or mislead-ing information (e.g. to suggest or let him assume he is not as ill as he is) is to lie to her patient, which is clearly wrong.

The only exception to this comes from another aspect of the doc-tor/patient relationship – the patient's assumption that the doc-tor will always act in his best interest. If a situation were to arise where it is clearly in his best interest not to tell a patient the truth (or the whole truth) then an exception could be made. But the onus is on the doctor to show, at least to her own satisfaction, that this is indeed the case.

The principles don't change when one is dealing with children or minors, though the fact that one is dealing with a child must be taken into account. First the parent or guardian must be fully involved. The intention should still be to tell the truth, but only to the extent that the child can cope with it or comprehend it, and this will depend both on the child and on the news. The overriding principle still remains to act in the best interest of the patient.

In this whole area it is important to remember that the doctor's relationship is with the patient, even though his next-of-kin, rel-atives and friends are also involved. This means that the doctor must tell the patient first, not a relative, and should only tell a relative with the patient's permission. This permission is often given implicitly. A husband may indicate that he wishes his wife to be included and involved, often by the simple fact that he brings his wife with him to some consultations. Alternatively, a doctor may tell a close relative serious or bad news in order to make it easier to tell the patient; e.g. it might be easier on the pat-ient if his wife is present when he is told his illness is terminal. Again, that's an example of the overriding principle of acting in the best interests of the patient.

What the doctor must avoid at all costs is allowing control of telling the patient to pass to a relative by disclosing information to a relative first in such a way that the relative can say 'Don't tell him; I don't want him to know', thus putting the doctor in an unenviable position. It is also a form of betrayal by the doctor of the relationship of truthfulness with her patient.

Breaking confidentiality

No person exists in isolation. Each is a part of society and each has responsibilities as well as rights in that society. One of those basic responsibilities is not to threaten or risk the lives of others. This fact can be the basis for a breach of medical confidentiality in certain exceptional circumstances.

For example in many countries the law obliges doctors to notify the police of any gunshot wounds they may treat. This is to establish that no one's life is in danger from criminal activity involving guns. Some very infectious diseases which are life-threatening may be listed as 'statutarily notifiable diseases', which means a doctor is obliged to report any instance of such a disease she may come across in order that infection may be controlled and lives protected. Most people would regard evidence or suspicion of child abuse as imposing an obligation to report it so that it can be investigated further. In some exceptional cases a judge may rule that in the interests of protecting society medical confidentiality must be broken, often by ordering access to medical records or obliging doctors to testify.

All of these are instances of the general principle that we have a basic responsibility to others in society to protect their right to life and not to endanger it unnecessarily. Exceptional cases may arise where this responsibility clashes with one's right to medical confidentiality, and in those cases the moral obligation weighs on the side of breaking confidentiality if there is no alternative.

Points for discussion or reflection

1. 'Conscience is the voice of God within us.' Do you agree?

2. Some argue that the instruction 'and proceed' on a consent form is much too general; others say that it is a sensible addition. How specific do you think such consent should be?

3. Discuss the extent to which the wishes of relatives should be respected in the care of the terminally ill patient.

4. Since all crime affects society in some degree, shouldn't a doctor report all evidence of crime to the authorities? If not, how do we establish the limits?

Notes:

1. J.F. Childress and J. Macquarrie (eds), *A New Dictionary of Christian Ethics*, p 116.

2. This issue arises again in the context of the use of children in clinical research. See chapter 8.

CHAPTER 3

The Definition of Death

We have already seen[1] that there is no one criterion for deciding that someone is alive. In ordinary usage we work with a long list of criteria, any one of which is usually sufficient – movement, communication, the ability to feel pain and so on, are all used. In borderline cases where the issue is more problematic, breathing, pulse and reaction to external stimuli become relevant criteria. Until quite recently these were the criteria for determining death, and are still used in most cases by the medical profession before a death certificate is issued.

However with recent medical developments these criteria have become problematic in certain situations. Life support systems can artificially maintain breathing and circulation of the blood when the patient is unable to do so. The purpose is to carry the patient through a difficult stage when he is unable to maintain breathing and circulation for himself and when without the support he would have died, through to the point where he is able to perform these functions for himself again. But what happens if the patient does not pull through? If breathing and circulation of the blood are the criteria for death, is not withdrawal of the support to be equated with causing the death of the patient? The development of organ transplants, especially more recently of the heart, where it is necessary to maintain circulation of the blood after death of the donor has occurred, placed further pressure on the demand to find a new and more appropriate set of criteria for determining death.

The Harvard criteria

This issue was addressed by a committee of the Harvard Medical School in 1968 and its opinion was published in the *Journal of the*

American Medical Association in that year. The committee was composed of ten physicians, a historian, a lawyer, and a theologian. It summarised the issue facing it thus:

> From ancient times down to the recent past it was clear that, when the respiration and heart stopped, the brain would die in a few minutes; so the obvious criterion of no heart beat as synonymous with death was sufficiently accurate. In those times the heart was considered to be the central organ of the body; it is not surprising that its failure marked the onset of death. This is no longer valid when modern resusitative and support measures are used. These improved activities can now restore 'life' as judged by the ancient standards of persistent respiration and continuing heart beat. This can be the case even when there is not the remotest possibility of an individual recovering consciousness following massive brain damage.[2]

The committee recommended that death should be understood in terms of 'a permanently non-functioning brain', but pointed out that this does not involve a denial of the traditional criteria, but recognises that additional criteria are needed for the new situations. The committee's criteria are complex, but have been summarised as '(1) unreceptivity and unresponsivity to externally applied stimuli and inner need; (2) absence of spontaneous muscular movements or spontaneous respiration; and (3) no elicitable reflexes. In addition a flat (isoelectric) electroencephalogram was held to be of great confirmatory value for the clinical diagnosis.'[3] In addition, that summary of the Harvard criteria added the following comment: 'Although generally referred to as criteria for 'cerebral death' or 'brain death', these criteria assess not only higher brain functions but brainstem and spinal cord activity and spontaneous respiration as well. The accumulating scientific evidence indicates that patients who meet the Harvard criteria will not recover and on autopsy will be found to have brains which are obviously destroyed, and supports the conclusion that these criteria may be useful for determining that death has occurred.'[4]

These criteria were quickly accepted worldwide as providing a safer set of criteria for determining that death has occurred in situations where traditional criteria had proved inadequate. Up to the 1960s it had not been possible to sustain breathing and circulation artificially. The cessation of either the lungs or the heart was automatically followed within minutes by the cessation of the other, and death of the brain through lack of oxygen.

Life support systems meant that the functioning of these organs could be separated. If the lungs or the heart ceased spontaneous functioning, ventilation or circulation could be maintained artifically, thus avoiding the death of the brain. Furthermore, again because of medical technology, doctors now had access to information on the functioning of the brain previously unavailable.

One of the reasons why brain-death criteria were accepted so readily was that they moved the criteria beyond the traditional criteria. Before the technology became available, the patient concerned would have been dead anyway – now the frontier had been extended, and the criteria were merely trying to catch up with the changed situation.

Paul Ramsey put all this into context. Brain-death criteria, he said, 'are proposals for updating our procedures for determining that death has occurred, for rebutting the belief that machines or treatments are the patient, for withdrawing the notion that artificially sustained signs of life are in themselves signs of life, for telling when we should stop circulating and ventilating the blood of an unburied corpse because there are no longer any vital functions really alive or recoverable in the patient'.[5]

The Karen Quinlan case

If the absence of brain activity is sufficient criteria for establishing that death has occurred, is the converse true? Is the presence of brain activity sufficient criteria for saying that the person is alive?

To address this question we need to look at a very famous court case in the United States in 1976 – the Karen Quinlan Case. Karen was a 22-year-old who for no apparent reason collapsed while out with friends. She was taken to hospital, but had already ceased breathing for at least two 15-minute periods. Within days it was apparent she was in a very deep coma, had suffered very severe brain damage, and needed a respirator to assist her breathing. Over time it became apparent that Karen's case was 'hopeless', and that there was no possibility of her emerging from the coma. Yet, because brain-death had not occurred, her doctors were unwilling to remove the respirator which it appeared was all that was keeping her alive. Eventually her father applied to the court to be made her guardian with the express power to authorise the withdrawal of the respirator.

The decision of that court is very important for that way we view death, because here was a person, not brain-dead, but in a very real way 'hopeless'. The fact that she was not dead was based on the Harvard brain-death criteria. The medical experts were 'satisfied that Karen met none of the criteria specified in the [Harvard] report and was therefore not "brain dead" within its contemplation'.[6] The medical evidence at the hearing described her as being in a 'chronic vegetative state', which was defined by one expert witness as a 'subject who remains with the capacity to maintain the vegetative parts of neurological function but who ... no longer has any cognitive function'.[7] Further, no form of treatment which can cure or improve that condition is known or available. As nearly as may be determined, considering the guarded area of remote uncertainties characteristic of most medical science predictions, she can never be restored to cognitive or sapient life'.[8]

The basic question before the court was, given all this evidence, was it morally acceptable to withdraw the respirator and allow this person to die?

Her father, a Roman Catholic, sought the opinion of his church prior to going to court, and, unusually, that advice was introduced at the hearing. It argued that one was not morally obliged to continue the use of artificial respiration in cases where the patient is completely hopeless – to withdraw such support is in no sense to be equated with euthanasia. 'Therefore the decision of Joseph Quinlan to request the discontinuance of this treatment is, according to the teachings of the Catholic Church, a morally correct decision.'[9]

The court went along with that opinion. It concluded that if all responsible medical opinion agreed 'that there is no reasonable possibility of Karen's ever emerging from her present comatose condition to a cognitive, sapient state, the present life-support system may be withdrawn and said action shall be without any civil or criminal liability'.[10]

These court proceedings were important because they expressed and clarified a number of issues which are generally recognised. To answer the question with which this section began: Is the presence of brain activity sufficient criterion for establishing that a person is alive? The Quinlan court opinion reveals a complex answer to that apparently simple question. Clearly, though she was in a persistent vegetative state, she was not dead. Because of this her doctors had introduced the respirator. They felt they could not accede to her father's request to withdraw the respirator because that would have caused her death.

The court, however, took seriously the fact that she was 'hopeless', and that there was no possibility of her ever returning to a cognitive, sapient state. Earlier (in Chapter 1) we saw that the 'ordinary language' meaning of being alive includes the capacity to relate, either to oneself, to others, or to the environment around us. This is very similar to the court's phrase, a 'cognitive, sapient state'. It was the absence of the potential for such a state, or, to express it differently, the absence of the potential to relate, that made all the difference to Karen. By agreeing to her father's request to enable him to have the respirator withdrawn, the court was recognising that Karen's life was ending, and that she was into the process of dying. The respirator was simply prolonging that process. Its withdrawal wouldn't cause her death; it would simply allow it to happen.

Death as a process

The Quinlan case has introduced us to an aspect of death and dying which is sometimes forgotten – the need to accept that a point may be reached when death is inevitable and must be accepted. Karen Quinlan was deeply comatose and a lot of time was taken over the decision as to what treatment was appropriate in

such a situation. What may surprise many is that there was any
real doubt as to the way to proceed. It would be assumed that
when a person is hopelessly ill then the form of treatment would
take account of that fact. A useful criterion in this area which has
been offered is that 'the use of any means should be based on
what is commonly termed a "reasonable hope of success"'.[11]
Perhaps the only quibble which could be raised against this is to
ask what is meant by 'success' in this context? The danger is that
'success' might be equated with recovery or an improved quality
of life. 'Success' in the management of the dying may mean 'en-
abling a comfortable or contented death'.

That aside, however, 'reasonable hope of success' does protect
the patient who is dying from unnecessary forms of treatment
which serve only to prolong the process. That concept might
have helped those involved in the management of Karen
Quinlan to think more clearly about how to proceed. It would
also help those involved with terminally ill patients to assess the
various treatment options available. The alternative is a type of
rule-book medicine where treatment is dictated by the nature of
the condition without regard to the needs of the patient.

A question which this whole discussion raises is whether we can
any longer speak of 'the moment of death'. Death is a process
with various stages. Death can be instantaneous as in a road traf-
fic accident, but more often today it stretches over a period of
time. For those around a bedside, a last breath marks the end.
Life support systems have divided the process up even more,
removing pulse and breathing as visible signs. Brain-death is a
significant point since it marks the end of that process; it marks
the end of any possibility to relate in any sense. The Quinlan
case demonstrated that we do not always have to wait for brain-
death to recognise that life is over. The potential can be absent
before brain-death and further medical treatment will serve
only to extend the dying process.

Some conclusions

Earlier in the chapter we saw that in ordinary usuage 'being
alive' is a complex notion, using a number of criteria, any one of
which would establish that a person is alive. These were sum-

marised in the phrase 'ability to relate'. When these criteria are absent (e.g. when someone is unconscious) we use spontaneous breathing and circulation (pulse) to establish that someone is alive. This is significant. Breathing and circulation indicate the *potential* to do all the things we regard as being alive. So it is not the *ability* but the *potential* to relate that is important. No one is suggesting that an unconscious person is any less alive than a conscious person. Life support systems have simply caused us to extend the criteria for assessing the existence of this potential to include criteria of brain activity.

An equally significant change is that *we now talk of death as a process, a process which ends with brain death, and within which the absence of any potential to relate marks a very significant stage and alters the sort of treatment we regard as appropriate.* The Quinlan case is important because it gave very public recognition to this. She was well into the process of dying, a process which would end with the death of her brain.

Incidentally, this discussion should help us dismiss one 'red herring' that is often raised in this context – cases of people who claimed to have 'died' and 'come back to life'. A common senario occurs in an operating theatre when the patient's heart stops for a brief period, and is then restarted. Given the discussion above it is simply incorrect to describe this situation as 'having died and then having been brought back to life'. Brain-death had not occurred – the potential to relate was not extinguished, as demonstrated by the patient telling the story! So too with 'out-of-body' experiences sometimes recounted from similar situations, either seeing the operating theatre including oneself from afar, or bright lights and celestial music. However else they may be explained, they cannot have been experiences or intimations of death, because if the patient is alive to tell the story then death cannot have occurred.

Organ transplants

Some comment should be made on the issues raised by the use of organs from recently deceased persons for transplant. In fact this practice was one of the factors pushing for a refinement of the criteria for defining death, since this is crucial for knowing when organs can be removed. Now that many of the technical problems associated with transplant surgery have been largely overcome (especially the problem of rejection) the demand for organs has grown enormously.

An important aspect of the technique is the necessity for the organs to be removed as soon as possible after the death of the donor. Patients on life support systems, for whom the brain-death criteria are often the most relevant, are often the very patients whose organs are most suitable for donation. It is possible to see a potential conflict which might arise between the care of a patient who is obviously dying and whose organs are suitable for donation, and the needs of another patient desperately in need of a transplant.

The normal response to the possibility of this clash of interests is to recommend that two separate medical teams be involved, one with each patient. The one concerned with the dying patient should manage and care for its patient without regard for the prospects for transplant, and should pronounce death by the appropriate criteria in the usual way. Only when death has occurred should the transplant team become involved.

Such a recommendation is obviously very wise. It avoids the possibility of a double standard arising in care for the dying – one standard for situations where a transplant is in prospect, and another when it is not. Almost as important is the clear division of responsibility between the two medical teams which enables the general public to have confidence on a very sensitive issue, and should encourage future potential donors.

We've already noted that the development of transplant surgery was partly responsible for encouraging the modern discussion of the definition of death. However, as Paul Ramsey points out, one must not allow the needs for transplant organs to determine or influence the criteria for determining death. It would be quite unacceptable to argue that because of the needs of transplant surgery we ought to alter our criteria for death to make more organs available or more usable because of earlier removal. 'If no person's death should for this purpose [i.e. transplant surgery]

be hastened, then the definition of death should not for this purpose be updated, or the procedures for stating that a man has
died be revised as a means of affording easier access to organs.'[12]

Points for discussion or reflection

1. Do you expect medical developments in the future to cause us
to reject the Harvard criteria of brain death in favour of more
adequate criteria? Why?

2. If you had been Karen Quinlan's doctor, what time of death
would you have entered on her death certificate? Why?

3. Must we always await brain death before declaring that death
has occurred?

4. Suppose a new technique for organ transplantation required
an organ to be removed pre-mortem, thus causing the death of
the donor, who knew this and had given consent and was close
to death himself. Could this be justified ethically?

Notes:
1. Chapter 1.
2. 'A Definition of Irreversible Coma', in the *Journal of the
American Medical Association* (1968), quoted in D.J. Horan and D.
Mall (eds), *Death, Dying and Euthanasia* (Maryland, 1980).
3. A.M. Capron and L.R. Kass 'A Statutory Definition of the
Standards for Determining Human Death: An Appraisal and a
Proposal', in *Death, Dying and Euthanasia*, pp 42-3.
4. ibid. pp 43-4.
5. P. Ramsey, *The Patient as Person* (Yale,1970), pp 88-9.
6. 'Opinion of the New Jersey Supreme Court in the Karen
Quinlan Case', in *Death, Dying and Euthanasia*, p 497.
7. ibid.
8. ibid. p 498.
9. ibid. p 503.
10. ibid. p 521.
11. P. Ramsey, op.cit., p 132.
12. ibid. p 103.

CHAPTER 4

Euthanasia

Any discussion of euthanasia today usually begins by pointing out that the word itself literally means 'easy death' or 'gentle death', something with which we would all agree and would probably seek for ourselves and for others. However the modern discussion has moved on considerably from these roots and now refers to decisions taken either to allow a seriously ill patient to die or to take steps to bring about that death. Though occasionally used (often very emotively) in others situations, which are in effect forms of suicide, we shall confine the discussion here to the context of the appropriate care of those who are dying, where each party involved – the medical staff, next-of-kin and the patient – is acting in good faith and genuinely wishes to do the best for the patient and those around him.

We must begin by making a crucial distinction between passive (or negative) euthanasia, and active (or positive) euthanasia: *Passive euthanasia* can be described as the withholding of medical treatment which would prolong the life of the gravely ill, usually because such treatment would effectively only prolong the process of dying; *active euthanasia* refers to deliberate action to end the life of the patient, often at the patient's request.

Passive euthanasia

A useful way into this aspect of euthanasia is to examine three different situations and consider an appropriate way to respond to each.

a. The irreversibly comatose patient

In previous chapters[1] we saw that it is the potential or the ability to relate in some way, however minimal, to oneself, to others and to the environment which is the basis of the respect we accord to human life. In the case of an irreversibly comatose patient, the ability to relate is at a low level and, because it is irreversible, the potential for any improvement is absent. The patient is well into the process of dying and further medical intervention can do nothing to reverse that process; it would merely serve to prolong dying and is not in any real sense sustaining human life. There is therefore no moral obligation to continue with medical intervention, other than to make the patient as comfortable as possible. Such was the case with Karen Quinlan discussed elsewhere.[2]

b. The conscious terminally-ill patient

There may come a point in the treatment of the terminally-ill patient when it is clear that further medical intervention will do little to extend his or her life and may even result in a diminution of the quality of life for that person. In such a situation freedom from pain, the ability to move about, to talk, and so on will assume greater value than active treatment of the condition in order simply to prolong life.

This approach is entirely consistent with our understanding of human life already discussed. Life is the ability or potential to relate and in situations where a condition is terminal, values associated with relating take on even greater value. The ability to relate to one's family and friends, to be in familiar places rather than a hospital ward, to be conscious, to be free of pain, and so on, become priorities. These priorities in care remain even if it becomes apparent that an unavoidable consequence may be that death is actually hastened by some of the treatments involved (e.g. the use of some very powerful pain-killers). In a very real sense the amount of life, measured in qualitative and not just quantitative terms, is increased by allowing a much greater degree of freedom to a terminally-ill patient as an alternative to pointless and wearisome medical intervention which might prolong life for an extra few days or weeks.

Ordinary and extraordinary means – a note: Before looking at the third situation it might be useful to consider a distinction sometimes made in this context between ordinary and extraordinary

means as a way of establishing which treatments are appropriate and which are not in the situations discussed. *Ordinary*
means what is well-established and regarded as normal within
the context in question; it is what we might expect a reasonable
person to undertake and offers the possibility of real benefit to
the patient. *Extraordinary* is anything which doesn't fit into this
criterion.

Which treatments are designated ordinary varies according to
the situation. Kidney dialysis might be ordinary in a city in
Western Europe or the United States; it might not be in rural
parts of Africa. An antibiotic to control pneumonia in an otherwise healthy young person would be ordinary; it might be inappropriate for someone well into the process of dying. Heart
transplants would be extraordinary means today; they might
not be twenty years hence.

The decision as to whether something is ordinary or not is made
from the perspective of the patient. Is it reasonable for a patient
in this situation and with this knowledge to refuse this particular treatment? Is it reasonable for the patient to expect that treatment be made available to him? Normally it is assumed that
there is a moral obligation on a patient to accept and for those
around him to provide 'ordinary' health care therapies, but that
'extraordinary' means carry no such obligation.

This distinction can be helpful in clarifying the discussion of
passive euthanasia. There is a moral obligation on medical staff
and the community in general to provide, and for the patient to
accept, 'ordinary' treatment which will be of genuine benefit to
the patient. There is no moral obligation to provide, or for the
patient to accept, 'extraordinary' treatment which in another
context is routine, but which for the dying patient merely pro-
longs existence and is in a real sense pointless.

c. The patient who refuses life-saving treatment

The distinction between ordinary and extraordinary means is
helpful in clarifying some of the moral issues involved in this
third situation. A patient may be advised that a particular course
of treatment is required to save his life; despite that advice the

patient refuses the treatment and discharges himself from hospital. His action is generally agreed to be unreasonable. The treatment concerned is 'ordinary' in the sense already defined – it offers reasonable hope of being of real benefit to the patient and is what one would expect a reasonable person to accept.

Two different sets of questions are raised – one for the doctor, the other for the patient.

We have already seen that the doctor has a moral obligation to offer this 'ordinary' treatment, but where lies this obligation if the patient refuses treatment? More basic than the obligation to make reasonable treatment available is the doctor's obligation to respect the personal integrity of her patient. Part of that integrity involves the concept of autonomy, which acknowledges that each person is a free moral agent with the right to exercise that freedom. It includes the right to make decisions about oneself and the right not to have things done to oneself without one's consent. Any person therefore has the right to refuse any treatment, and no one may force medical treatment on anyone else, no matter how necessary or desirable that treatment may be for the life or well-being of the patient. The doctor then has fulfilled her obligations if she has made the treatment available and has honestly and clearly explained the implications of the treatment and the consequences of refusal to the patient.

For the patient a different set of questions arise. These centre on the reasons for his refusal, and they may range from (a) a considered decision not to undergo painful and debilitating treatment with only a fair chance of success, to (b) effectively making a decision for suicide.

If (a), the distinction between ordinary and extraordinary can be of help once again. We've already seen that the categorisation of a treatment into ordinary or extraordinary is made from the patient's perspective. A 'reasonable' patient may decide that a particular treatment which others regard as ordinary, or perhaps borderline, is for him 'extraordinary'. The possible benefits are outweighed by the discomfort and pain involved, perhaps treatment would limit him freedom to talk or move about, or involve unacceptable risk. Others may disagree with the patient but still accept his decision and after some discussion would recognise it as a morally responsible decision of a free agent.

If, however, the refusal is more of the second type, type (b), a different moral approach is required. If the refusal is unreasonable, i.e. the proposed treatment offers the prospect of genuine benefit (in all senses) to the patient, and without it he will die, then it is tantamount to a decision for suicide. So the question becomes: do we have a moral right to opt for suicide?

A moral right to commit suicide?

Most arguments against suicide are religious and we shall look at them, but first we will look at some of the secular discussions of the subject.

Secular arguments: Most secular arguments against suicide centre either on one's responsibility to oneself or to society. Each person, it is argued, has certain duties to himself. The list of such duties varies considerably depending on who one is listening to but it often includes a duty to seek happiness, to avoid pain, to respect one's bodily integrity (e.g. against unnecessary self-mutilation), self defence, and to preserve one's life. This last duty is often seen as primary because without it no other duty makes sense. An act of suicide, it is argued, is a deliberate act against this primary duty, and so is fundamentally wrong.

This argument is relevant for the situation we have been considering – the patient who unreasonably refuses treatment – but is questionable in other contexts. These questions centre on the making the duty to preserve one's own life a primary duty owed to oneself, which gives a value to human life over all other principles. But against this, many would say that the deaths of martyrs and heroes who gave their lives for a higher principle are admirable, unless we want to say they were always misguided. Is not an anti-war protestor who covers himself in petrol and sets himself alight standing for a principle which he regards as higher than his own life? So, it is argued, preserving one's own life is not always a primary duty – there can be values higher than this.

David Hume, the eighteenth century philosopher, put another argument in favour of suicide: 'Suppose that it is no longer in my power to promote the interest of society; suppose that I am a burden to it; suppose that my life hinders some person from being more useful to society: in such cases, my resignation of life must not only be innocent but laudable'.[3] This is a form of utilitarian argument, based on the usefulness or otherwise of a particular individual to society. However we must ask: in the end of the day is usefulness to society the only or even the final measure of a person's value and worth?

A strong response to this type of utilitarian argument can be made by arguing that relationships are what give a person value. Peter Baelz (a Christian theologian) mentions one such argument:

> ... in human relationships there are 'canons of loyalty' which should guide our moral decisions, and ... these may be more fundamental than the utilitarian is prepared to admit. The texture of our common life is made up not only of utilitarian considerations, but also of covenanted relationships which are held to be good in themselves and to be the expression of our fundamental humanity. To call attention to these relationships does not immediately answer the moral question concerning suicide. It does, however, put it in a somewhat different light.[4]

Baelz is very tentative in introducing this style of argument, but others are more forthright. One such is Germain Grisez who makes very clear his reasons for condemning any act of suicide:

> Even if suicide in some cases does not conflict with any specific duty which a person has to others, it does terminate one's capacity for community. A person who separates himself from his own bodily life takes the last step in what is usually a long process of withdrawal from intimate communion with the world and with other persons. One who commits suicide breaks off relations definitely; he does not go gently and reluctantly from our midst, but leaves willingly, as it were slamming the door as he departs. The shock is bound to upset those who are left behind.

Moreover, each individual who willingly abandons the project of human life in community makes it more difficult for others to carry on. This is especially so for others who are discouraged. Each fresh example of self-destruction compels many sensible people to think once more about the unthinkable. Thus, one who commits suicide bequeaths his own misery to others and intensifies their suffering.[5]

Religious arguments: The direction of these secular arguments brings us close to some of the religious arguments against suicide, for if non-religious arguments can use the fact that relationships are basic to our existence and impose obligations on us, then even more so will Christians, whose faith is rooted in relationships, use similar arguments.

First we should note that the Bible itself contains no specific condemnation of suicide. In fact in the Old Testament Samson's action in bringing down the Temple and thereby causing his own death is portrayed as praiseworthy (Jdgs 16:30), and in the New Testament, as Baelz points out 'even the suicide of Judas, if such it was (but *cf* Acts 1:18 with Mt 27:5) is not explicitly condemned. It was his betrayal of Jesus rather than the manner of his death which constituted his grave sin and evoked the real horror'.[6] However, nothwithstanding these and other very exceptional cases (e.g. the deaths of martyrs) the whole tradition of Christianity has been against suicide in all but the most exceptional cases.

Christian arguments against suicide usually fall under one of the following categories:

a) Life is a gift from God as creator, and to deliberately take one's own or another's life is a rejection of that gift and an act of rebellion against God;

b) Each human life is special because it reflects the image of God, no matter how marred that image may appear to be. This status, conferred on each person at creation, entails responsibilities as well as privileges. One of these responsibilities is always to treat all human life including one's own as special, because all reflect God's glory. Obviously, with such a view of human life, suicide can never be right.

c) The third type of argument is a development of the secular 'relationships' argument already discussed. Persons do not live in isolation – they exist in community and in relationships with others. For a Christian those relationships include a relationship with God. To take one's life, then, is not just an action for the individual. It always affects others and alters one's relationship with God (even though Christians believe that one can continue to have a relationship with God after death). Suicide, if you like, is a unilateral action which closes or alters basic relationships for oneself and for others. It always causes deep pain and so is morally wrong.

The question 'do we have a moral right to commit suicide?' then admits of no easy answer. The initial argument in its favour, that we each have a right to self-determination which includes the right to decide to end one's life, has had responses from both secular and religious sources. In the final analysis, it is up to each person to assess the value and validity of these arguments and to make up one's own mind on the morality of suicide.

The fact that many countries have now removed suicide from the sanction of law does not alter the moral questions surrounding suicide. Repeal of laws outlawing suicide does not imply that suicide is now acceptable, it is simply asserting that it is inappropriate to use the law in this area, though it almost always remains an offence to assist another to commit suicide.

Also, the above discussion has ignored the fact that very many suicides or potential suicides are suffering from a psychological illness or considerable psychological distress. In such situations the patient cannot be assumed to be open to rational argument or even clear reflection about the morality or otherwise of what he or she is proposing to do.

This discussion of suicide arose out of consideration of a patient's decision to refuse life-saving treatment. We have seen that such may be a reasonable decision to refuse to undergo painful and debilitating treatment which offers little prospect of success – effectively the patient has decided that the proposed treatment was 'extraordinary' and so was under no obligation to pursue it.

At the other end of the spectrum, that patient's decision may be quite unreasonable and inexplicable to those around him, and be tantamount to a decision for suicide.

From the doctor's perspective the issues are clearer. Her obligation is to respect the autonomy of her patient and abide by the patient's decision to refuse treatment, and to provide whatever ease and comfort she can and is allowed to.

Dying with dignity

It is common today to remark that death has replaced sex as the great taboo in modern society. It is one subject no one wishes to discuss; we dislike being in the presence of death and the dying, and we avoid contact with the necessary trappings of death.

Death is often protrayed as a battle, to which we must bring the armour of medicine and the weapons of modern technology, and it is easy for the medical profession to accept this role. Huge advances in medicine have done much to prevent unnecessary or untimely death, but death is still the great inevitable in life and no amount of scientific advances will alter that.

The language we use reflects our attitudes. We talk of the fight for life, and significantly we describe someone who has accepted the inevitability of his own death as 'having lost the will to live'.

The examples discussed in this chapter focused on circumstances where we must accept the inevitability of death and that further medical intervention will do little for the dignity of the person concerned. The three cases involved the withdrawal or refusal of treatment and the situations where this is morally acceptable. Finding an appropriate point to withold further treatment and allowing death to occur is what is properly meant by the phrase 'dying with dignity', and the hospice movement has been to the fore in putting this philosophy into practice. By accepting that some conditions are terminal and that the emphasis of medical care in such cases should be on comfort and pain control, that movement has recovered the old concept of a 'good death' and of a 'gentle' or 'easy death'.

Active euthanasia

The particular form of active euthanasia we will consider is when a patient suffering from a terminal illness requests his doctor to end his life. Such a request is not just for the withdrawal of life-sustaining treatment; it is a request that the doctor take steps to end the patient's life – the most common way is by the use of a lethal injection, or by providing a prescription for a lethal dose.

In most jurisdictions this is illegal, though there is pressure in a number of countries for this to be changed. Two situations where this pressure has already resulted in changes in the law are the state of Oregon in the United States and the Netherlands.

Oregon: In a suprise judgment in May 1994 a court in Oregon ruled that a doctor may assist a terminally ill patient to commit suicide. The case had been brought by three patients and five physicians who treat terminally ill patients, and also by an organisation called Compassion in Dying, which provides support, counselling and assistance to terminally ill patients considering suicide. The judgment concluded that 'a competent, terminally ill adult has a constitutionally guaranteed right under the 14th amendment to commit physician-assisted suicide'[7]

The 14th Amendment 'is essentially a direction that all persons similarly situated should be treated alike'.[8] It was argued in court that 'under current state law, those terminally ill persons whose condition involves the use of life-sustaining equipment may lawfully obtain medical assistance in terminating such treatment, including food and water, and thereby hasten death, while those who also suffer from terminal illnesses, but whose treatment does not involve the use of life-support systems, are denied the option of hastening death with medical assistance.' 'The court finds the two groups of mentally competent, terminally ill adults at issue here to be similarly situated.'[9]

The argument here is important. What is implied is that a terminally ill patient who is dependent on medical assistance to support his life has the option of committing suicide simply by refusing treatment; therefore a terminally ill patient who is not so dependent should have the right to seek medical assistance in committing suicide, on the grounds that he should have equal rights with the other patient. But is this so?

We have seen that any patient has the right to refuse treatment, even if this is tantamount to a decision for suicide.[10] However, a doctor's compliance with this refusal is rooted in her respect for the right of any individual not to have treatment forced on him against his will. It is not based on a doctor's respect for her patient's right to commit suicide.

We also saw[11] that from a patient's perspective the refusal of treatment may represent a considered decision not to undergo painful and debilitating treatment which, if he is terminally ill, offers no long term prospect for success. This was described as a morally responsible decision of a free agent. On the other hand the refusal of treatment may be unreasonable and inexplicable to those around him, and so may amount to a decision for suicide.

It appears that the Oregon Court decided that *all* decisions by terminally ill patients to refuse treatment were primarily decisions to opt for suicide, and the recognition of the right to refuse treatment was interpreted as a recognition of the right to commit suicide, at least for the terminally ill. This is clearly not the case. The right to refuse treatment is rooted in the concept of autonomy, not in the right to commit suicide.

Because of this court judgment, the issue of physician-assisted suicide was put to the people of Oregon in Ballot Measure 16 in November 1994, and approved. The measure permits terminally ill patients to obtain a prescription for lethal drugs from their doctor. Such patients must be mentally competent and their death must have been predicted to occur within six months. Each patient must have made at least three requests (two oral and one written) for such a prescription over a 15 day period. The doctor is expressly forbidden to administer the dose herself – it must be self-administered by the patient.

From the patient's perspective, the moral questions centre on the morality of suicide, already discussed.[12] However, more complex are the questions posed to the doctor. First, there is the doctor's own attitude to suicide, since she should not be obliged to participate in a procedure with which she disagrees. If her own personal morality allows for suicide as an option in some situations, there is the further question whether she should co-operate in a particular patient's suicide. Is this patient making a genuinely free decision in opting for suicide? Though Measure 16 specifies counselling if it is believed that the patient has a mental disorder or impaired judgment from depression, and confirmation from another doctor that the patient is capable of acting voluntarily, these determinations are notoriously difficult to make with any degree of certainty. Further, it does not allow for other pressures such as family pressures, the fear of being a burden, or the fear of a painful or undignified death. The fact that the measure makes some allowance for impaired judgment and depression is a tacit acknowledgement of the fact that a doctor cannot be certain of a free and voluntary request simply because the patient has repeated the request on a number of occasions.

The Netherlands: The situation in Oregon is akin to that in the Netherlands, but there is one very important difference – in Oregon a doctor may facilitate the suicide of a terminally ill patient by providing a prescription for a lethal dose, but may not administer the dose herself; in the Netherlands the doctor may, and usually does, administer the lethal dose or injection.

Strictly speaking active euthanasia is a criminal offence in the Netherlands, and this was re-affirmed in November 1993. 'Medical actions which accelerate the termination of life must be reported to the Public Prosecutor, who will decide on a case-by-case basis whether prosecution should follow.'[13] In practice, however, prosecution does not follow if certain strict guidelines have been followed. These are:
- the patient persistently has requested euthanasia,
- the patient is in a hopeless and intolerable situation,
- the physican has consulted another physician about the diagnosis and prognosis,
- the physican can provide a written report with all the relevant medical data about the disease and the death of the patient.[14]

These four criteria provide a useful outline for a discussion of active euthanasia, but from an ethical perspective the first two are the most important. The third (consulting another physican) is an important check on the doctor's diagnosis to rule out the possibility of error in diagnosis or prognosis; the fourth is necessary for the report to the public prosecutor.

The first, the patient's persistent request, embodies the notion of autonomy and self-determination discussed in Chapter 2, and this is the main argument offered in favour of active euthanasia. We know that each person has the right to decide what is and isn't done to him, and cannot have treatment forced on him against his wishes. This right, as we've already seen, includes the right to refuse treatment even if the patient will die as a consequence. One may question the morality of someone effectively committing suicide in this way, but this does not justify forcing treatment on that person against his will.

This principle of self-determination is being invoked again in the case of active euthanasia – however in this case the doctor is being asked to end the patient's life. We've already seen that the morality of suicide is very questionable; what is now being considered is whether the patient has the moral right to ask for euthanasia from his doctor, and whether the doctor has the right to comply with the request. From the patient's perspective, the request is effectively one for medical assistance in committing suicide; the morality of suicide has already been discussed earlier in the chapter where we saw that arguments from self-determination have had significant responses from both secular and religious sources. But should a doctor respond to such a request for assistance?

The administration of a lethal injection is contrary to all that the medical profession stands for. In the Hippocratic Oath there is a commitment to work 'for the benefit of the sick according to my ability and judgment', to keep them free from harm and injustice, and specifically a promise that 'I will neither give a deadly drug to anybody if asked for it, nor will I make a suggestion to this effect'. In response to this it could be argued that active euthanasia may, in certain circumstances, be for the benefit of the patient, if that patient has asked for it, and if the patient is in a 'hopeless and intolerable situation' (the second Dutch criterion). What would qualify as such a situation? The one most people think of and which is most often cited is a terminally ill patient in a situation of intolerable pain which cannot be controlled or alleviated. The question whether such a situation could arise in reality is a medical question, but there is a considerable body of opinion in the medical profession, especially among specialists in the area of palliative care, that with proper management no patient should ever find himself in a hopeless and intolerable situation because of pain. While this may be argued over by doctors and other specialists, there is a further question that if one believes that such situations can in fact arise, whether the introduction of active euthanasia is the appropriate response, or whether further development of pain management and pain control offers a more humane response?

The Tony Bland case

As a result of injuries sustained in the disaster at Hillsborough football stadium in Britain in 1989 in which ninety-five people were killed, Tony Bland had been in a 'persistent vegetative state' (PVS) for almost four years. His condition was described in a newspaper report: 'His limbs contorted, his eyes open with only their reflex causing movement, he has been kept alive by a tube passing down his nose and throat and into his stomach. He is unaware of his parents' presence or of the intensive nursing care at the Airdale Hospital which keeps down infections and prevents further shrivelling. The parts of his brain which provided him with consciousness have turned to fluid.'[15] His consultant was certain he had 'absolutely no chance of recovery'. The hospital authorities applied to the courts to establish if they might lawfully discontinue life-saving and medically supportive treatment designed to keep him alive in his permanent vegetative state. Eventually the Law Lords upheld that right in 1993, artificial feeding was discontinued, and Mr Bland died.

That decision caused considerable controversy at the time. Many welcomed the decision, others condemned it as a form of active euthanasia. There is no disagreement about the fact that Tony

Bland's case was 'hopeless' in the way Karen Quinlan was hopeless – for him there was no possibility of a return to a cognitive
sapient state either (see page 29 above). In the Karen Quinlan
case there was widespread agreement that it was inappropriate
to continue with the life-support system. Was not the Tony Bland
case the same? The main form of 'life saving and medical supportive treatment' (the Law Lords phrase) for him was the tube
supplying food to his stomach – there was no life-support system or its equivalent in use in this case, and so a few days after
the legal judgment this feeding apparatus was not reconnected.
His doctor said that this would not cause him to starve to death;
he would probably fall victim to an infection or kidney failure
before that.

Certainly Tony Bland's case was hopeless and so further medical intervention was pointless since it did not hold out the
prospect of improvement in his condition – at best it could only
prolong the process of dying for him. Where most of the controversy arose was over the means – discontinuing feeding – which
many found morally unacceptable. To this it was responded that
the means was irrelevant from the patient's perspective; using
the most immediate means simply helped shorten the agony for
his parents.

To understand why some found the means unacceptable we
should refer again to the distinction between ordinary and extraordinary treatment. 'Ordinary' means what is well established and regarded as normal within the context; it is what we
might expect a reasonable person to undertake and offers the
possibility of real benefit to the patient. 'Extraordinary' is anything which does not fit this criterion. Is a feeding tube 'ordinary' or 'extraordinary'? This question was at the heart of the
debate. In the context in question it offered no possibility of real
benefit to the patient (nor would anything else), yet feeding a
patient, even through a tube, is part of normal hospital routine.
Everyone would regard it as unreasonable for a hospital to
refuse to feed a patient, even one who is dying. It is here that the
unease arises. Most people regard feeding a patient, even in the
situation in question, as 'ordinary' even if medical means (a
tube) is being used, and so it was unreasonable to discontinue

feeding. However it would not have been unreasonable to continue feeding but if an infection developed, not to fight it with
antibiotics, which would amount to an extraordinary treatment
in this context.

The accusation that this was active euthanasia by another name
is harder to sustain. As we have already seen, there is a world of
difference, morally, between discontinuing treatment and taking steps to end someone's life by, for example, administering a
lethal drug.

This case is yet another example of the pressures on medical
practice, medical ethics and the law to keep up with the very
rapid developments we see taking place. The fact that such cases
can arise so unexpectedly and cause such controversy shows
how difficult it is for ethicists and lawyers to anticipate the next
area of debate, and for the discussion of them to get ahead of the
situations. What does appear certain is that the management of
death and decisions about appropriate care for the dying will
continue to be a central issue in medical ethics for some time to
come.

Points for discussion or reflection

1. Formulate your own answer to the question: 'Does a terminally
ill person have a moral right to commit suicide?'

2. Does the concept 'dying with dignity' have any real meaning
in the modern medical management of death?

3. Compare and contrast the situations in Oregon and the
Netherlands as outlined with respect to euthanasia and assisted
suicide.

4. Should the wishes of an unconscious patient expressed in a
'living will' always be respected? Should special conditions and
limits apply?

Notes:
1. Chapters 1 and 3.
2. See pages 27-29.

3. D. Hume, 'On Suicide' (1777), in *Hume on Religion*, (Fontana, 1963) p 260.

4. P. Baelz, 'Voluntary Euthanasia', in *Theology*, Vol LXXV No 623, May 1972, p 243.

5. G. Grisez, 'Suicide and Euthanasia', in D.J. Horan and D. Mall (eds), *Death, Dying and Euthanasia* (Maryland,1980) p 780.

6. P. Baelz, op. cit., p 239n.

7. *Origins*, May 26, 1994, Vol. 24. No. 2, p 17.

8. ibid, p 26.

9. ibid.

10. See pages 36-38.

11. ibid.

12. See pages 38-42.

13. Netherlands Ministry of Justice, Press Release, November 1993.

14. H.M. Dupuis, 'Euthanasia in the Netherlands: Facts and Moral Arguments', in *Annals of Oncology* 4 (1993), p 448.

15. *Independent* (London), 5 February 1993, p 2.

CHAPTER 5

Abortion

Few issues in medical ethics raise such emotions as the question of abortion. Feelings run high on either side; protests and marches either for or against abortion can still draw large numbers in some countries and have even on occasion led to violence. Against such a backdrop, it's difficult for anyone to decide the issue calmly for oneself, and also to understand the reasoning of those with whom one disagrees.

First we have to admit that when we look back in history at the issue there is no absolutely consistent approach to abortion, even within the Christian tradition. Virtually all theologians in early church history disapprove of abortion, though much of their discussion is concerned with the distinction between the formed and unformed fetus (i.e. the belief that there is a stage after conception when the fetus is 'formed' into a human person) and with the point of ensoulment (when the soul enters the body). St Augustine (the fifth century theologian) said that the fetus is ensouled at forty-six days, while St Aquinas (thirteenth century) followed Aristotle in saying that formation takes place at forty days for the male and ninety days for the female. Both regarded abortion as a very serious crime, but Aquinas only regarded it as homicide after formation. The Irish Penitentials used this distinction for grading their penalties: 'for the destruction of the embryo of a child in the mother's womb', three years on bread and water, and 'for the destruction of flesh and spirit [i.e. the animated fetus] in the womb,' fourteen years on bread and water'.[1]

However, while acknowledging diversity within the Christian tradition on the exact status of the fetus at different stages, we must remember that the Christian tradition, and consequently most of Western society, has traditionally condemned abortion. Also, most of the discussion within Christianity took place with a primitive understanding of the origins of human life and of fetal development which we know today to be simply false, and is very far removed from the issue of abortion as it confronts us today, with our vastly improved understanding of the process of conception and development within the womb. This modern understanding, though, has not served to resolve the moral questions involved – in fact if anything, it has served to polarise them.

Two typical statements may serve to illustrate this:

1) 'The Women's Liberation movement sees abortion as the most significant liberation of all, from the body and from male domination. The most effective solution to unwanted pregnancy, it removes the final block to full control of reproduction. Unless reproduction can be fully controlled, women will remain in bondage not only to their sexuality but, even more, to those legions of male chauvinists who use female sexuality to their own domineering ends.'[2]

2) Abortion indicates 'the kind of respect society will show the most defenseless beings in our midst. If the life of a defenseless fetus is not respected, then there is good reason to believe that the most fundamental of all human rights – the right to life – will have been subverted at its core. The test of the humane society is not the respect it pays to the strongest and most articulate, but that which it accords to the weakest and least articulate.'[2]

Not everyone will be able to identify fully with either of these statements, and many will see their own attitude somewhere between the two, but one basic issue divides these two statements from one another. The first statement speaks only of the rights of the woman – it sees abortion as concerning one person only. The second statement talks of two lives – the mother and the fetus. The difference between the two then centres on the status of the fetus (or embryo) – is it a person just like its mother, or is it (in the early stages at least) simply a part of a woman's body? The most basic issue we have to address then, is the status of the embryo.

The status of the embryo

While moral arguments about the status of the embryo are often complex and very divisive, it is possible I think to divide the current popular debate into three arguments. I shall call them the *continuity argument*, the *process argument*, and the *right to choose argument*. The first two start from the status of an adult person, and then proceed to ask 'when does this status begin?'

The continuity argument

What constitutes personal identity? I am a person, and I am the same person I was yesterday. How do I know? Because I remember being here yesterday, being married to the same person, living in this house, working at this job, etc. If pushed to provide proof that I am the same person who was here yesterday I could try to show all the intermediate places I have been since then – in other words to show that there is continuity in space and time between the person who was here yesterday and me today. I would try to show I am the same body, with the same thoughts, feelings, memories, etc.

The same could be done (in theory anyway) to show that I am the same person I was five or ten or twenty years ago. In fact my identity with the baby shown in a photograph in an album at home could be established by proving that that baby grew up to be me, so that I could say 'that's me at six weeks old', even though appearance, memory, thoughts etc. have all changed.

My identity stretches back to babyhood, to birth, and further back to the baby in the womb – how much further can we go back before that? In fact identity goes right back to the time when one sperm met one ovum. At that moment of conception an entity was formed which, despite numerous changes, became me. There is continuity between the fertilised ovum and the person we see today.

That entity (me!) is a person now. When did I become a person? There is nothing that happened to the ovum or later to the baby in its development, no stage it went through, which made it a person. The status of personhood must have been there from the very beginning.

An argument of this sort is often used by those who are opposed to abortion in any circumstances. For example it can be found in a Roman Catholic document on abortion: 'From the time that the ovum is fertilised, a life is begun which is neither that of the father nor of the mother; it is rather the life of a new human being with its own growth. It would never be made human if it were not human already',[3] though, interestingly, the document goes on to make a distinction between being a human being and being a person, and appears to allow for the possibility that we may not be dealing with a *person* from the moment of conception: '… it is not up to the biological sciences to make a definitive judgment on questions which are properly philosophical and moral, such as the moment when a human person is constituted or the legitimacy of abortion. From a moral point of view this is certain: even if doubt existed concerning whether the fruit of conception is already a human person, it is objectively a grave sin to dare to risk murder.'[4]

This argument leads to clear answers on the question of abortion – abortion is the killing of an unborn person, and therefore is always wrong.

The double-effect principle

This principle is often mentioned in conjunction with a firm anti-abortion stance, such as that just outlined, as a way of coping morally with two particular cases where termination of a pregnancy is unavoidable.

The principle is one most would readily accept. When we intend to do something which is good in itself, but the only way to achieve it is by doing incidental but unavoidable harm, it is still acceptable to do the action. For example, a lot of surgery in undertaken in the knowledge that it will cause the patient a degree of pain afterwards. It is acceptable to cause this pain if there is no other way of achieving the good intended by the operation. Situations like that can be multiplied in medicine and dentistry, but the principle does not only apply in the medical context. A parent may scold a child and thus cause upset 'for its own good'.

In the context of abortion, the principle is often invoked to defend two exceptions to a general anti-abortion approach: (a) an ectopic pregnancy (which is one which has begun in the fallopian tube) would threaten the life of the mother if allowed to progress. A doctor may treat it by removing the 'diseased' tube in order to save the mother's life, even though this will also terminate the pregnancy. The intention is to treat the diseased organ to save the woman's life; an unintended though unavoidable consequence of this is the death of the fetus. A particular moral difficulty for the use of the principle in this case is the medical possibility of removing the fetus directly and so leaving the tube intact (though perhaps damaged), thus removing the 'double effect' aspect of the treatment.

(b) A pregnant woman suffering from cancer of the womb may have have her womb removed as part of the treatment of the cancer, even though this has the unavoidable consequence of killing the fetus. The primary intention is to treat the disease; the unavoidable consequence is the termination of the pregnancy.

The process argument

Like the continuity argument, this one begins with everyday language. A person is an entity which thinks, talks, reflects, has memories, feels sensations, eats, walks, etc. Being a person does not imply the ability to do all these, but the absence of the capacity to perform any function such as these would cause most people to question whether in fact we are dealing with a person. A Church of England report summarised it well:

> At the foot of these powers [associated with being a person] is the phenomenon of consciousness, and it is as a subject of consciousness ... that we value the human being most fundamentally. It is important not to suggest that human beings must exercise some specific degree of intelligence or emotional maturity before they can properly be regarded as human persons. Yet, if we are to draw a morally relevant distinction between humans and other animals, we seem compelled to define the human in terms of a sort of nature able to exercise rational, moral and personal capacities. We need to assert that all members of this species possess such a nature, even where, through some impediment, it cannot properly be exercised in many particular cases.[5]

In order to be a subject of consciousness, to perform any of the functions we associate with persons, we need a functioning brain. We've already seen (see pages 25-27 above) that the absence of any brain activity is a sufficient criterion for determining that death has occurred. So the question of the beginning of life can be addressed by looking at the early stages of brain development.

The *Warnock Report*, which is the report of a commission set up in 1982 by the British Government to inquire into the whole area of human fertilisation and embryology, provides a useful summary of the various early stages of development of the embryo.[6] At fertilisation one cell is created, from which two, then four, eight, etc, identical cells are formed. This cluster of cells goes through a number of changes until the first recognisable features of the embryo proper appear (11.4). 'The first of these features is the primitive streak', and sometimes two primitive streaks may appear which means we have a case of identical twins. This is the latest stage at which identical twins can occur (11.5). This is, I think, a significant stage – the latest stage at which twins may occur, called individuation, and the first at which recognisable features of the embryo proper appear. This happens 14 or 15 days after fertilisation. Throughout all this implantation is taking place. 'There is a very high wastage rate ... as a result of [embryo's] failure to implant' (11.7). The emergence of the primitive streak marks the start of a period of very rapid change. 'By the seventeenth day the neural groove appears and by the twenty-second to twenty-third day this has developed to become the neural folds, which in turn start to fuse and form the recognisable antecedent of the spinal cord' (11.5). This marks the earliest stage of the appearance of something which will become the future brain.

The *Warnock Report* recommended that it was from the time of the formation of the primitive streak that protection should be afforded, since 'this marks the beginning of individual development' (11.22). The Church of England in its response to this report agreed with this position, and a later document pointed out that other points of embryonic development can be argued to be crucially significant also. 'For example, the establishment of a functioning nerve-net at around forty days after conception can be regarded as a necessary criterion for the beginning of personal life, paralleling the common acceptance of brain-death (as distinct from, say, heart-failure) as the mark of the end of physical life'.[7]

The Roman Catholic theologian, Bernard Häring, also sees merit in considering these early developments as having crucial significance. 'Can it then be said that at least before the twenty-fifth to fortieth day, the embryo cannot yet (with certainty) be considered as a human person? or, to put it differently, that only about that time the embryo becomes a being with all the basic rights of a human person? At the present moment, however, this is no more than an opinion which deserves serious consideration and further discussion.'[8] However he adds that he is not prepared to change his own position on abortion on the basis of a 'mere theory'.

While some may wish to choose one of these significant points as the point at which personhood begins, it is more common to use these successive stages as the basis of an argument that becoming a person is a process from conception to birth – a process which commands respect at each stage simply because it is the process of coming to life, and within which respect must grow as the embryo does.

The thinking behind this approach was, I think, well summarised by John Habgood, the Anglican Archbishop of York. 'Biological processes are not amenable to the sharp distinctions that lawyers like to make. It seems to me that the conceptus is neither simply a thing nor simply a person. It is an organism on its way to becoming a person ... The process of creation is a process of interactions going on during a period of development.'[9]

In considering this view we might look to our attitudes to natural miscarriages. For many parents, when a miscarriage occurs, especially in the later stages, there is a sense of having lost a baby, and that a death has occurred. On the other hand, if it happens in the early stages the feeling might best be described as a loss of hope, a sadness that what might have been will not now happen; it is not quite the same as a sense of a death having occurred. Of course we cannot generalise about the feelings of everyone, but if this distinction has any validity then it may reflect our deep emotional response to miscarriage, and different responses at different stages.

The process argument only ever sees termination of a pregnancy as a last resort, and requiring more and more serious justification as the pregnancy continues. The situations where it might be contemplated are always exceptional and will vary, but may include pregnancy after rape or incest, especially when the victim is young, the use of the morning-after pill in a sexual assault clinic, treatment of ectopic pregnancy or of cancer in any part of the body where delay would threaten the woman's life, situations where the pregnancy itself poses a serious threat to the life of the woman, or where severe abnormality in the fetus has been detected such that if born it would not survive. While such terminations are always regretted, they are not regarded as distruction of a human person when they occur in the early stages.

Is there a cut off point, a point beyond which a termination is unacceptable? To be consistent, we should look to brain-based criteria. The basic structure of the human cerebral cortex takes shape between the fifteenth and twenty-fifth day; there is a functioning nerve-net around forty days; by eight weeks there is detectable electrical brain activity; by twelve weeks the brain structure is complete. Those who look for brain-based criteria usually cite one of these stages (often the twelve-week stage) as the point beyond which termination is not morally acceptable.

'Right to choose' argument

A third approach argues that the decision whether or not to continue with a pregnancy is a decision for the woman concerned, and for her alone, since it is she who will have to carry the pregnancy and bear the child.

There are two important assumptions in this. One is that abortion is a necessary part of the full control of reproduction, and is therefore to be seen as related to contraception. The second is that the fetus has no separate status, especially in the early stages; it is simply part of the woman's body.

These assumptions are very questionable. Firstly, the decision not to proceed with a pregnancy which has begun (abortion) is substantially different from the decision to take steps to avoid becoming pregnant (contraception). Under any interpretation, there is a sense of destroying something in the case of abortion which is not present in the case of contraception. The right to full control of reproduction is an argument in favour of full access to contraception. There has to be a separate argument justifying its extension to abortion.

Secondly, the contention that the fetus is simply part of the woman's body is open to question. It is an obvious biological fact that it is in the woman's body, but it doesn't thereby follow that it is part of her body in the way that liver, arms and heart are. The fetus has a separate genetic constitution and grows and develops independently of the woman, though dependent on her. These facts alone should indicate a separate status for the fetus.

These arguments do tell against the idea that abortion is simply a matter for the woman concerned, but do not imply that any pro-abortion argument is therefore untenable. A stronger moral basis for such an argument may be to argue that the fetus does not acquire the status of a person until late in the process of coming to birth, and that it is the woman's choice up to then. This is implicit in British abortion legislation, where 'viability' (the capacity for independent existence) is the criterion. The original legislation of 1967 marked twenty-eight weeks as the limit beyond which a termination could not be performed, and this was recently modified to twenty-four weeks because recent medical advances have brought viability forward to this stage.

This stage (twenty-four weeks) was also chosen in United States legislation in 1973 as the latest stage for a termination, though states are free to choose an earlier stage as the limit. Interestingly the Supreme Court avoided the question of whether life begins at this point. 'We need not resolve the difficult question of when life begins. When those trained in the respective disciplines of medicine, philosophy and theology are unable to arrive at any consensus, the judiciary ... is not in a position to speculate as to the answer.' Elsewhere in the decision they point to viability as the decisive point: 'With respect to the states' important and legitimate interest in potential life, the compelling point is at viability ... State regulation protective of foetal life after viability has both logical and biological justification.'[10]

This agreement in the legal context on viability raises some questions. First, it does not represent agreement on the beginning of the person (as the American Supreme Court explicitly stated). In fact viability represents the latest stage at which a termination would in any sense be acceptable to any reasonable person. Very few would hold that one should end the life of a baby who is capable of living – in such a case the issue would have shifted from abortion to infanticide – but the fact that few if any would accept abortion after this point does not imply that most would accept it up to this point.

Secondly, the determination of viability can change with medical progress, as in the change in Britain from twenty-eight weeks to twenty-four weeks. However the most fundamental objection must be the basis on which viability is seen as crucial. Viability is the point at which the fetus could live outside the womb. However, as Bernard Häring has pointed out, 'the fact that it cannot survive outside its natural habitat does not allow one to deprive it of its life-saving environment'.[11]

Some conclusions

We have seen that the status of the embryo is central to the morality of abortion, yet this is the issue which is most divisive. I have outlined three different arguments, and there are very many more, and many variants on them.

Viability does not address the question of the status of the embryo at all – in fact it can be seen as the maximum position, beyond which one might, morally at least, be accused of infanticide. The process argument, using brain criteria, has the distinct merit of mirroring the modern discussion of the determination of death (see chapter 3), where brain criteria are also used. The morally safest position is the continuity argument, and many favour it simply because some doubts exist over other theories. On the other hand, many find questionable the implicit attribution of personhood to a cluster of cells.

Some related issues

Abortifacients: The ethical debate about contraception dominated the 1960s, and at that time it was common to make a moral distinction about the way different forms of contraception operated. Some suppress ovulation (e.g. 'the pill'), some prevent sperm and ovum from meeting (e.g. condoms), others act after sperm and ovum have met by preventing implantation of the fertilised ovum in the womb (e.g. the IUD), while others, notably the 'morning after pill', either prevent implantation, or if implantation has occurred, dislodge it.

Those which act after conception, such as the 'morning after pill', were called by the loaded term 'abortifacient', and some ethicists who accepted the morality of contraception still objected to abortifacient forms of contraception. I say the term 'abortifacient' is loaded, because it literally means 'making (or causing) an abortion', and that is exactly the ethical question which has to be answered.

The answer is implicit in the discussion of abortion. If we believe personhood should be attributed at conception, as in the continuity argument above, then forms of contraception which act after conception (abortifacient) will be unacceptable. If one accepts a later date for personhood (as in the process argument) then all forms of contraception including post-conception contraception are morally acceptable.

The morning-after pill: This is one of the issues raised by the use of the 'morning-after' pill, taken after coitus has taken place. It acts by causing a shedding of the lining of the womb (in the form of a heavy period), thus preventing a fertilised ovum from implanting in the womb, or if it has already implanted, causing it to be flushed off the wall of the womb. It is often used as a form of late contraception, and routinely offered to victims at sexual assaults clinics. When used as a form of late contraception the moral questions are no different from the use of any other form of post-conception contraception already discussed (though there may be medical concerns since the dosage is often quite toxic), but the issues are more complex when used by victims of sexual assault, and it is on this use that the discussion will centre.

First, let us deal with one common moral fallacy. It is not uncommon to hear the argument that moral questions do not arise with its use, since at the time of its use one does not know if the victim has conceived or not. This is plainly a bad argument. While it is true one does not know, it is certainly the intention to prevent a pregnancy. If conception has taken place the pregnancy will be stopped; if no conception has taken place then the drug was unnecessary.

For victims (and those who care for them) who accept the use of abortifacient contraception there are no added moral difficulties with the use of the morning-after pill. The difficulty arises only for those who argue that personhood must be attributed at conception. One can obviously argue that a new life may have begun and that, no matter what the circumstances of its origins, it must be allowed to go to full term, even though this will probably be traumatic for the victim.

However it is also possible to argue that because of the violence of the assault, and because of the lack of any form of consent on the part of the victim, there is no moral obligation on her to carry the pregnancy through to term. It can be argued that one is faced with a dilemma: either the victim has to allow the pregnancy to proceed, with all the emotional trauma that that entails; or the pregnancy should be ended. In such circumstances one is literally faced with a choice between two evils, and the judgment as to which is the lesser of the two must be decided by those involved. One has to balance the destruction of the fertilised ovum against the emotional and psychological destruction of the victim if the pregnancy proceeds. In such circumstances a person who otherwise might reject the use of abortificient forms of contraception might find the morning-after pill acceptable in some cases of sexual assault.

The abortion drug: Mention must also be made of the development of the 'abortion drug' RU486, developed in France. Trials have been conducted in several countries and it has been licenced for use in France where it is widely available, and more recently in Britain. There is considerable debate about its efficiency but it is likely that these difficulties will be overcome in due course.

No new moral questions of principle about abortion are raised by its availability, but moral concerns do centre on the fact that it 'privatises' abortion, so that the prospect of not needing to refer to a registered clinic at all is raised. In turn this means that the woman may well avoid proper counselling, and also the waiting time, which provides an opportunity for reflection, is removed. Also, while it may be possible to control its use by licencing in Western countries, a greater concern may be its indiscriminate use in third world countries without proper medical super-vision, which is more than likely.

Abortion is a very emotional issue, and one sad aspect of the whole debate is the frequent unwillingness of many to counten-ance the sincerity and moral integrity of those from whom they differ. In this chapter a number of issues and aspects have been left open-ended so that one may decide the issue for oneself, and also take the opportunity to try to understand the thinking and perspective of those from whom one differs.

Points for discussion or reflection

1. State your own opinion on the status of the embryo at various stages of development.

2. To what extent does the double effect principle address 'diffi-cult cases' in the area of abortion?

3. In legislating for abortion, the US Supreme Court avoided the question of when life begins. Does this question *have* to be an-swered before legislating on the subject?

4. Examine the moral and social implications of the widespread availability of the abortion drug (RU 486).

Notes:

1. N. Anderson, *Issues of Life and Death* (Norfolk Press,1976) p 77.
The original document dates from the eighth century.

2. D. Callahan, 'Abortion: Some Ethical Issues', in T.A. Shannon
(ed), *Bioethics*, 2nd ed, (Paulist, 1981), p 13-14.

3. *Declaration on Procured Abortion* (Sacred Congregation for the
Doctrine of the Faith, 1974), paragraph 12.

4. ibid, paragraph 13.

5. *Personal Origins: The Report of a Working Party on Human
Fertilisation and Embryology of the Board for Social Responsibility*
(Church of England), (CIO, 1985), paragraph 89.

6. *The Warnock Report: Report of the Committee of Inquiry into Human
Fertilisation and Embryology* (1984), paragraphs 11.2-11.7

7. *Personal Origins*, paragraph 88.

8. B. Häring, *Medical Ethics*, 3rd ed, (St. Paul, 1991), p 79.

9. J. Habgood, quoted in *The Independent* (London) 8 February
1990, p 2.

10. Quoted in D. Brown, *Choices* (Blackwell,1983), p 117.

11. B. Häring, op. cit., p 90.

CHAPTER 6

Assisted Conception

In 1978 Louise Brown became the first baby to be born by in-vitro fertilisation (IVF), a process which is popularly called 'test tube babies'. Her birth was a cause for celebration not only for her parents but also for many thousands of childless couples throughout the world, for it opened the possibility of medical help for certain categories of childlessness.

It was a technique which also raised many questions, and these and other related issues were examined by a commission of inquiry set up by the British Government to investigate this whole area. Popularly known as the *Warnock Report*, after its chairperson Dame Mary Warnock, it reported in 1984 and was widely circulated and discussed throughout the world. Though it does not really address ethical aspects of the various techniques in any depth – its brief was to make recommendations for legislation and regulation – it serves as a useful introduction to the many aspects of the techniques available to assist or enable conception.[1]

The techniques

All of the techniques discussed in the *Warnock Report* aim to assist couples overcome a medical problem which prevents them having children in the normal way. They are:

Artificial insemination by husband (AIH): When for some medical reason a couple cannot conceive through normal intercourse, it may be possible to take semen from the husband (or partner) obtained by masturbation, and insert it under clinical conditions into the woman's womb at the appropriate time in her cycle, in the hope that she will conceive. It can be used, for example, when a man has a low sperm count, which makes conception unlikely. Semen can be collected in this manner on a number of occasions and inserted at one time into the woman's womb, thus making conception more likely.

Artificial insemination by donor (AID): If the husband is unable to produce any sperm at all, then it is possible to use sperm from a donor. When medically supervised there is usually screening for genetic defects in the donor, and also a limit is placed on the number of times a person may donate.

In-vitro fertilisation (IVF): The breakthrough that Louise Brown's birth represented was the successful fertilisation of an ovum outside the mother's body. In IVF an ovum is removed from the woman's ovaries, mixed with sperm from her husband in a test-tube, and, if fertilisation occurs, the fertilised ovum is replaced in the woman's womb and the pregnancy continues as normal. The technique is very useful, for example, if a woman's fallopian tubes have been damaged or removed (e.g. by previous ectopic pregnancies).

This brief account, however, conceals the fact that the chance of success at each stage is very low, and it may be necessary to make repeated attempts in order to achieve a successful pregnancy. According to the *Warnock Report* (5.2-5.4) the chance of success is considerably enhanced if a number of fertilised ova are used (the ova are obtained by use of a drug which causes superovulation in the ovaries) so that a number can be transferred to the womb in the hope that one will implant successfully.

In-vitro fertilisation by donor: As with artificial insemination, what is possible between partners is also possible with ova from a donor, if for example the ovaries have been damaged. From the donor's perspective donation is more difficult since it involves a minor operation to remove the ova, but sometimes a woman undergoing another operation, e.g. a sterilisation, may agree to take a drug to cause superovulation and to have those eggs removed for donation at the same time.

Surrogacy: If a medical problem means that a woman is unable to carry a pregnancy to term, it is possible to remove her ovum, mix with semen from her partner, and if it fertilises, to place it in another woman's womb who then carries the pregnancy, and at birth return the child to the original couple. In this case the child is genetically related to the original couple, but not to the woman who was pregnant and gave birth.

At this stage it might help if we clarified some of the terminology surrounding parenthood in this context, since our usual words 'mother' and 'father' can mean different persons in various contexts.

I will use the term *genetic parents* or *genetic mother* or *genetic father* to refer to those who provide the ovum or sperm from which the child results. I will call the woman who carries the pregnancy and gives birth the *physiological mother*, and those who are the socially accepted parents i.e. those who rear the child, *social parents*. We should also note that we already accept a division in parental roles in the case of adoption, where the genetic parents and physiological mother are different from the social parents.

I will also limit the discussion to cases of assisted conception which are medically determined, i.e. where there is a medical reason why a child cannot be conceived or born in the usual way, and so I am excluding cases where, for example, a film star is unwilling to interrupt her career to become pregnant and so seeks the help of a surrogate mother to carry her child; or where a couple wish to use donated sperm or ova simply because they want certain genetic characteristics for their child, e.g. to be blond or tall. I will also assume the technique is under proper medical supervision.

Some ethical issues

Artificial insemination by husband (AIH): Few ethical questions are raised by the use of this technique but some are raised by conservative Christians. One centres on masturbation which is the method used to obtain the semen. Some early Christian writers condemned masturbation as being on a par with abortion, because it was believed (mistakenly) that semen contained the whole human offspring, with the woman simply providing a suitable environment in which it can grow. It is still condemned in official Roman Catholic teaching on the grounds that it is a misuse of the reproductive organs, no matter what the purpose. 'Whatever the motive for acting in this way, the deliberate use of the sexual faculty outside normal conjugal relations essentially contradicts the finality of the faculty.'[2]

A further argument against AIH appears in a later document from the Vatican.[3] Most people would accept that sexual inter-course has at least two functions: the physical expression of love between two people (the unitive aspect), and as the usual means for conceiving a child (the procreative aspect). When discussing the morality of artificial contraception, official Roman Catholic teaching argued that the unitive and procreative aspects cannot be separated; both must be present on each occasion of sexual intercourse,[4] hence the opposition to artificial contraception. The same argument is applied in the later document to AIH, be-cause it separates procreation from sexual intercourse. 'Artificial insemination as a substitute for the conjugal act is prohibited by reason of the voluntary dissociation of the two meanings of the conjugal act'; if, however the technique is used to facilitate the procreative aspect of intercourse (and not to replace it) 'it can be morally acceptable'.[5] While this grudging acceptance of AIH represents official teaching, it is only fair to point out that many Roman Catholic moral theologians defend the technique more vigorously, arguing that since it takes place within the totality of marriage and since the purpose (having a child) is good, AIH is morally acceptable when no other option is available.

Apart from these questions, there are no substantial objections to the practice of AIH, which most see as a useful technique for dealing with some causes of infertility.

In-vitro fertilisation (IVF): Though from a medical perspective IVF is a far more complex procedure, from an ethical point of view at its simplest it is very similar to AIH. In both cases the technique is attempting to overcome a difficulty in conception, though in the case of IVF the assisted conception takes place out-side the woman's body in a laboratory. So if one accepts AIH one can usually accept the principle underlying IVF; if AIH is unacceptable then IVF will also be unacceptable.

However, few things in medicine are ever simple, and there is an important extra element to IVF. This is well summarised in the *Warnock Report*: Because of difficulties in achieving a successful implantation of the fertilised ovum in the uterus,

> ... it is common practice to transfer more than one embryo to the potential mother whenever possible, and for this reason several eggs need to be recovered. This is achieved by artificial stimulation, known as superovulation, of the woman's ovaries to ensure that she produces several eggs in one cycle. After an appropriate course of drugs, as many ripe eggs as are accessible are harvested just before the time of ovulation. Each egg is then mixed with semen to achieve fertilisation. Assuming there is no abnormality in the semen, the success rate of fertilisation is usually at least 75%. Some embryos may however show signs of poor or abnormal development; when the time comes to transfer the embryos to the woman it may be that there is only one embryo suitable for transfer, or there may be several. (5.3)

There is obviously no problem when there is only one, or even two. But what if there are more, more than can be safely transferred into the uterus, given the significant hazards to both mother and babies associated with multiple pregnancies? What can we do with the spare embryos? One possibility is to freeze them, so that they can be used if the current attempt is unsuccessful or used for a subsequent pregnancy. But what if they are not required? Can we let them 'die', or destroy them? The word 'die' is placed in inverted commas because its very use presupposes an answer to the fundamental question in this area – what is the status of an embryo at this stage?

This is the same question as was raised in the discussion of abortion (page 53), and the answer is far from clear. We saw, when looking at abortion, that there is a variety of answers to that question, among which the continuity, process and right to choose arguments are the most important. For those who hold to the continuity argument, the creation of spare embryos, i.e. embryos which will not be implanted in the uterus, is wrong for the same reason that abortion even at the earliest stage is wrong – because it is the deliberate ending of a human life.

The process argument differs substantially from this. While it is unclear as to when personhood should be attributed, it is also clear that it should not be attributed in the early stages, and certainly not before the 15-25 day stage. As such, the spare embryos issue in IVF do not present a particular moral problem, nor are there moral difficulties for those who regard viability as the significant stage (the right to choose argument).

The involvement of donors and third parties

In the case of both AIH and IVF so far discussed, the genetic parents (those from whom the semen or ovum come) are the same as the social parents (those who rear the child). All that has happened is that medicine has helped overcome a difficulty in achieving conception. However, what can be done within a couple's relationship can also be achieved with semen or ova from an outside donor, usually someone unknown to the couple. A donor can be used when one or other of the couple is unable to produce gamete material (semen or ova). Many who find artificial insemination and IVF otherwise acceptable object when donors are used.

So what specific ethical issues are raised by the use of donated material? I think it is possible to simplify many of the moral arguments into two approaches – there are those who see the use of a donor as akin to adoption, and those who see it as a form of adultery.

In adoption, the genetic parents are unable or unwilling to rear the child they have conceived, and so another couple undertake to become the child's social parents and take responsibility for the child. With adoption the needs of the child for social parents are matched with the desire of a couple for a child.

It is possible to see artificial insemination by donor (AID) or IVF by donor as one stage better than adoption. With adoption, neither social parent is genetically related to the child; with AID donated semen is used so the social father is different from the genetic father, but the genetic mother carries the baby and is the social mother. This is better than adoption because one parent at least (the mother in this case) is genetically related to the child and has also carried the pregnancy. The father's position is akin to an adoptive father.

So too with IVF by donor. Here a donated ovum is used. The social father is also the genetic father, and the social mother, though not genetically related to the child, has had the satisfaction of carrying the pregnancy. Again it appears to be a stage better than adoption.

The similarities with adoption are obvious, but there are also differences. The most obvious is that in adoption the primary concern is with the child and its need for social parents. These needs are met in a way that also meets the desire of a couple for a child, but the needs of the couple are not central. It would not be acceptable for example to encourage women to become pregnant simply to provide children for adoption. On the other hand, with AID and IVF the central concern is with the needs of the couple and that is a very big difference, though of course the needs of the child are not ignored.

Those who see the use of donors in such techniques as a form of adultery argue that the procreation of children is an important component of marriage or life-long relationship. To use a donor in procreation is to introduce a third party into a marriage relationship in one of its most central aspects (having children). To conceive a child by the used of donated semen or ova is akin to conceiving a child through an affair with a third party. It is a form of adultery.

However, there is one obvious difference. With AIH and IVF by donor there is no personal relationship or involvement with the donor. Usually the couple never meet or know the donor, and having a child may even strengthen and confirm the couple's relationship. If it is to be seen as a form of adultery, then it can only be so in the most technical sense.

Because there is such a huge gap between the way different people approach assisted conception by the use of donated material, the attitude of the couple seeking such help is vital. It is possible for partners to see the issue very differently, and this may cause problems for their relationship at some stage. In particular there is a danger that the partner who cannot produce gamete material will perhaps unconsciously feel left out of the process even though he or she has agreed to it, and may harbour deep-seated feelings of resentment towards the future child. For these reasons most agree that serious counselling should be undertaken by both partners before a technique involving donated material is embarked on, so that each may fully understand his or her own feelings on the issue and also those of the partner.

Embryo donation: If it is possible to use either donated semen or donated ova it is also possible to use both at the same time, for example when neither partner can produce gamete material. In this case a donated ovum is fertilised with donated semen in vitro, and then placed in the womb of the woman seeking the child. The child will not be genetically related to either social parent, but the woman has carried the pregnancy.

As a technique it is exactly the same as IVF and raises the same moral questions. Two donors are involved instead of one, and as such it brings us a stage closer to adoption – in fact it is sometimes called pre-natal adoption. If one can accept the practice of IVF and the use of donated material then it is difficult to support a moral objection to embryo donation in situations where it is medically determined.

Surrogacy: Surrogacy, which is when a woman carries a pregnancy for another couple and then 'hands over' the baby at birth, has been seen to raise serious moral questions, and these have been compounded by the great emotional difficulties which are often encountered.

The moral questions centre on the fact that another person, an 'outsider' to the relationship, is being introduced into the family situation in a very real and personal way. The surrogate mother is carrying a baby to whom she is not genetically related and whom she will not rear. This will involve her emotionally with the couple whose child it is during the pregnancy, but also and at least as important, she is emotionally involved with the baby she is carrying. Society has only recently become aware of the relationship between a woman and the baby in pregnancy which we call *bonding*, but it is now recognised as very important to both woman and baby.

Such emotional involvement is fraught with problems for all concerned and for this reason there is general condemnation in moral circles of the practice of surrogacy. This is supported by stories, often reported sensationally in newspapers, of surrogate mothers who are reluctant to give the baby to the genetic parents at birth. Court cases over the issue have also occurred. Such highly publicised cases are only the public side of many less well-known but equally emotional situations for both parents and surrogate mother. The law is still very unclear in this area, and is probably an inappropriate instrument for resolving emotional issues such as this. The ethical condemnation centres on setting out to create situations which, while motivated by altruistic concern for a childless couple, can lead to such emotional conflict and turmoil for all concerned.

Throughout this whole discussion of assisted conception, we must be careful not to treat a baby as though it were a product – something to be produced in the most efficient and effective manner – and forget that we are dealing with what will become a person with all the needs and rights associated with personhood. We must also be wary of talking about a 'right to have a baby'. A baby is a gift – religious people describe it as a gift from God – and all agree that having a child is a privilege and a great responsibility. Medical technology can now enable some hitherto childless couples to have children, but this should not lessen our sense of respect for the privilege of parenthood, nor our wonder at the miracle of new life.

Translating that into practice may be more difficult, since the possibility of some techniques usually leads to demands for its use in situations which were not envisaged at the outset. We will look at some of these in the next chapter.

Points for discussion or reflection

1. Do parents have a *right* to have a child?

2. Do moral questions arise for donors of gamete material used in medically assisted conception?

3. How does adoption differ from assisted conception by donor?

4. Are there situations where surrogacy would be morally acceptable?

Notes:

1. *The Warnock Report: Report of the Committee of Inquiry into Human Fertilisation and Embryology* (1984). It has already been referred to in Chapter 5.

2. *Declaration on Certain Questions Concerning Sexual Ethics* (Sacred Congregation for the Doctrine of the Faith, 1975) paragraph 9.

3. *Instruction on Respect for Human Life in its Origins and on the Dignity of Procreation* (Congregation for the Doctrine of the Faith, 1987). This document also discusses IVF, the use of donated gamete material, and research on embryos.

4. *Humanae Vitae: Encylical Letter of Pope Paul VI,* (1968), paragraphs 11 and 12.

5. *Instruction on Respect for Human Life,* p 10.

CHAPTER 7

Assisted Conception: Some Related Issues

As we begin to look briefly at some further possibilities with assisted conception it is useful to remind ourselves that the purpose of medicine in this area is to assist nature to overcome medical difficulties and to remedy natural deficiencies. A useful parallel might be the involvement of medicine in sport. We accept medical assistance and the use of drugs in overcoming injuries and developing potential, but not the use of drugs to enhance performance beyond what could naturally be achieved. Practices which go beyond this, e.g. attempts to create superhumans in sport, are seen as morally wrong and an abuse of nature. This is why at the beginning of the previous chapter the discussion was limited to situations which are medically determined – where there is a medical reason why a child cannot be conceived or born in the usual way.

Issues in parenting

The above point will help in approaching some of the new possibilities which are now available in parenting and making some brief comments on them.

Lesbian Parents: We often hear of requests by lesbian couples to have a child by IVF. Many issues are raised by this possibility – the most common argument against it being that a child needs to grow up in an environment where there is both a male and a female parent, to which the response must be that many children grow up in homes where there is only one parent, or there are only two women (say, the mother and an aunt), and do not obviously suffer because of it. A child's main need is for love and security and this is not guaranteed by having a man and woman as parents, nor is it excluded because both parents are women.

The question really is: should medicine support this possibility by providing IVF treatment in such cases? It seems to me that medicine should be very reluctant to become involved in such a practice since it goes beyond the accepted sense of assisted conception, and is not a situation which could ever occur naturally.

Procreating after death: We often hear of court cases where a widow attempts to establish ownership of her late husband's semen which had been frozen and stored in a clinic before his death. The purpose of this is so that she can have a child by artificial insemination. Such cases usually centre on the question of ownership, but there is a separate moral question as to whether medicine should be involved in this practice even if it were legal.

Again we know the pattern in nature that at death one loses all possibility of procreating, and it would seem to follow that medicine should not be involved in going beyond nature in this way. It would be logical then for all stored semen to be destroyed on the death of the donor.

Post-menopausal mothers: It is not a defect in nature when a woman ceases to be able to have children after menopause, so it would appear to be a misuse of medicine to use it to create a situation which could not occur naturally, in this case by the use of hormone or other therapies. The fact that a man can father into old age does not seem to me to be a counter argument.

Research on embryos

Techniques such as IVF emerged after long years of medical research, and are still being improved and developed. An issue which arises is whether embryos could be used in such research. The prospect is one which often evokes an immediate sense of revultion, so let us be clear about what exactly is being proposed before making a judgment.

What is proposed is that under certain conditions embryos, either those left over as part of the IVF technique or specially created for the purpose, be used for genuine research purposes either of a general kind or specifically to improve IVF techniques, up to the fourteen-day day stage. It is obviously not intended that the embryos should have the possibility of life after the research.

For those who say that life begins at conception, such research will obviously be unacceptable, in the same way that creating spare embryos as part of IVF is unacceptable.

Those who take a different view about the beginning of life (e.g. the process approach) may be open to the prospect of research under certain conditions. The issue becomes one of respect, which in the end must be a subjective judgment. While one may not be prepared to say that the embryo is a human person, certainly not in the early stages, there must be a degree of respect due to it because it has the potential for human life. That in turn becomes the question of how one expresses that respect.

Some will argue that respect demands that no such research be undertaken. This was a minority view in the *Warnock Report*,[1] which also went on to argue that respect also demanded that that in IVF no more embryos than it was possible to use should be created during the process. Others have argued that spare embryos produced as part of IVF treatment may be used for legitimate research purposes, but it would be wrong to create embryos specifically for research. Yet others hold that the good intended by the research overcomes any sense of disrespect which may be perceived by their use, and so genuine research for worthwhile purposes is permitted and the creation of embryos for this purpose is acceptable. This latter was the argument of the *Warnock Report* (11.18). In *Personal Origins*[2] it is argued that any of these options might be held by a Christian.

One common feature of all who would accept some research on embryos is the view that research must be worthwhile and necessary, and so would see strict licencing and regulatory control over all such research as essential. Also research is only permitted up to the fourteen-day day stage, when the embryo is still a microscopic cluster of cells and individuation has not taken place (see page 56 above).

Donated ovarian tissue – a possibility?

In such a fast developing field it is almost impossible to speculate as to what will be the next ethical question to arise in this area, but the Human Fertilisation and Embryology Authority in

Britain issued a public consultation document in 1994 entitled *Donated Ovarian Tissue in Embryo Research and Assisted Conception*, which opened up for discussion an issue which it felt would arise in the near future.

It centres on the source of ova for use in IVF treatment. The number of donors is limited because it involves taking a fertility drug and a minor operation each time. Often it is women who are undergoing sterilisation who agree to donate or those who are undergoing IVF treatment themselves and have spare ova. The number of ova available is not sufficient for the demand and the waiting lists for treatment are very long.

The document envisages that within a short period it may be possible to take ovarian tissue from a number of sources, including adult donors, those who have died (as with kidney, heart and other transplants already) and from aborted fetuses. All could be sources of immature ova, which could be matured in vitro, and also ovarian tissue could be grafted into a recipient woman, thus making her fertile. Apparently there are millions of immature ova in fetal ovaries and thousands still remaining in the normally fertile woman which have the potential to ripen into mature eggs. The advantages of such sources of ova becoming available for IVF treatment, for research, and for dealing with infertility by grafting are obvious. While these remain only possibilities for the future, it is obvious that if they do become possibilities there will be very considerable ethical controversy over their use.

I think it is fair to say that most people feel considerable unease about the possibility of these developments, but it is worthwhile asking ourselves what *ethical* questions are raised and how we respond to them. What follows can only be my own response, but it may serve to introduce the topic for others.

In my opinion a central ethical issue is that of consent by the donor, so let us consider the various categories of donor from that perspective.

1) *Adult donors:* The donation of any tissue or organ by any living adult can only be done with the clear consent of the person

concerned. However, the donation of any human tissue with the possibility of reproducing raises even bigger issues. The capacity to reproduce is bound up with what we are as individuals and imposes a relationship of some sort between the donor and the future child. At minimum there is a genetic relationship since the donated material will determine in part at least the genetic make-up of the child. If we accept the practice of AID and IVF by donor (this was discussed in the previous chapter) then I believe we should be prepared to accept the donation of ovarian material by a consenting adult as envisaged in the document. However, in the existing case of AID and IVF the donor knows what is happening and has consented to each case of donation, and the same should apply when donating ovarian material. Separate and specific consent in full knowledge of the facts should be obtained from the donor on each occasion of donation. The general existing guidelines for AID and IVF donation with respect to screening, confidentiality, access to information etc, should also apply.

2) *Donation after death:* Again the main issue is that of consent. After death the right to consent to the donation of organs (e.g. kidneys, heart, etc) rests with the next of kin, though the wishes of the deceased are usually respected, but ovarian tissue cannot be treated in the same way, for reasons stated in the previous paragraph. There is a relationship between the donor and the child which doesn't exist with heart or lung donation.

Yet do we wish to say that the sort of donation envisaged should always be forbidden? In my opinion, it would be legitimate to consider that a person before death, fully understanding all the issues involved, could give specific permission for such donation after death. Because of the nature of the donation, such permission could not be assumed within a general consent to donate organs (e.g. in a general organ donor card), nor could it be open to next of kin to give such consent.

3) *Aborted fetuses:* If the procedure as envisaged were to occur there would be a genetic relationship between the donor fetus and the future child. While there would also be some genetic relationship between the mother of the fetus and the future child it

would be at one remove and therefore more distant (as a child to one of its grandparents). Law and morality do not confer rights and responsibilities on grandparents for their grandchildren, so it is difficult to see how a mother of an aborted fetus could give consent with respect to possible offspring from that fetus. If consent can't be given by her, by whom then can it be given? For this reason I would be opposed to the use of fetal ovarian tissue in this way.

There is considerable controversy about abortion already. If one regards life as beginning at conception then one will find any use at all of fetal tissue unacceptable. Alternatively, if one sees personhood as something gradually acquired one will still wish to talk in terms of appropriate respect for the fetus. 'Appropriate respect' is a matter of judgment, but for many any use of fetal tissue for treatment or research does not fall within this category, and even more so the use of ovarian fetal tissue for treatment or research is not 'appropriate respect'.

Points for discussion or reflection

1. Would consent by the donor before death alter the moral issues surrounding procreation after death?

2. Outline your own position on the use of embryos in research.

3. The discussion of donated ovarian tissue in the chapter centred on the question of consent. Are other moral questions involved?

Notes:
1. *The Warnock Report: Report of the Committee of Inquiry into Human Fertilisation and Embryology* (1984), Expression of Dissent B.
2. *Personal Origins: The Report of a Working Party on Human Fertilisation and Embryology* (1984), paragraphs 132-9.

CHAPTER 8

Medical Research

The progress of medicine, like the rest of scientific development, depends on research. Ideas are developed, theories are explored, but in the end each new drug or therapy has to be tested. The first stage of the testing can often take place in the laboratory; sometimes animals are used for tests, but before a new drug or technique can be released for general use it has to be tried on human beings. Sometimes research needs information along the way which can only be obtained from human beings. If progress is going to be made, human beings will have to be used as test subjects in clinical research in some way or other.

A minimal sense of research

The most common form of clinical research is so common that we often do not recognise it as such. This is where a doctor tries a different form of treatment on a patient to see if it is more effective – if not she may switch back to the original treatment. Such practice hardly counts as research since the new treatment has been well tested, side effects are known and it is in general use. It is a form of research since the doctor is trying the treatment out and testing it on a particular patient to see if it suits. The primary intention of course is to improve the treatment of the patient, not to test the drug.

A related form of research might be better described as experience. There is an element of uncertainty and risk about all medical treatment; patients react in different and sometimes surprising ways so that no one can predict the outcome with absolute certainty, and it could be said that experience with previous patients is part of research in that sense. Such research is incidental to the routine work of medicine in treating illness, and provided the research does not become a purpose for the treatment, few ethical questions are raised.

A different form of research arises when the medical records, family histories and lifestyles of patients are scrutinised to establish a common factor or combination of factors which may give a clue to the origin or cause of a particular disease. Indications of the causes of certain forms of cancer (e.g. the relationship between smoking and lung cancer, or the effects of asbestos) and of AIDS have been established in this way, and the current interest in environmental influences on health many uncover many more connections.

All such are forms of research which are so common that we take them for granted and seldom give rise to ethical debate.

Controlled trials

The type of formal research we are most familiar with is experiments with forms of treatment where the effects of treatment are uncertain. It is the testing on human subjects after all other tests have been completed to establish a track record for the treatment and identify any side-effects and so on; all of which must be done before the treatment is made available to the general public.

The most popular way to do this is through the use of controlled trials, where a group of people is identified, half are given the treatment and the others are not. The larger the group the more accurate will be the results, since people and their illnesses vary considerably and it can often be difficult to know if they are getting better or not, and whether any improvement is due to the treatment or whether they would have improved anyway. A larger group produces greater statistical accuracy – how large depends on the nature and importance of the research at that particular stage.

At one time it was not uncommon for such trials to be done retrospectively. A group of patients were simply given the proposed treatment routinely by their doctors and the effects then compared with the general body of patients, but as a way of testing a treatment today this is quite unacceptable. The element of risk associated with any new and untried treatment alone should raise ethical questions since it is no part of the ethos of medicine to put a patient's life or health unnecessarily at risk.

Therapeutic and non-therapeutic trials

When discussing clinical trials, a distinction is usually made between therapeutic and non-therapeutic trials. Therapeutic trials are where the patient suffers from the condition, and the research aims to establish a new or modified treatment which is likely to be or is expected to be at least as good if not better than the existing treatment (if such exists) and so there is a possibility of direct benefit to the patient if he agrees to become a test subject. Non-therapeutic trials are those where research results are the only purpose – the test subject is not expected to benefit medically from the trial himself.

In both types of trials it is always assumed that the risk to the subject has been reduced as much as possible by testing the treatment in a laboratory and on animals to establish as far as possible the likely effects and side-effects, and to ensure the safety of the subject.

Therapeutic trials fall into two classes. The first is where no treatment for the condition exists. To eliminate other factors from the trial it is common to use placebos – drugs or tablets which look, taste, etc, exactly like the active treatment but which are ineffective – which are administered randomly to some among the group, while the rest are given the new treatment. To make certain that no hint is given as to who is getting the active treatment and who is getting the placebo, a double-blind can be used, where neither the patients nor the researcher dealing directly with them knows who is getting what, and a more complex set of records is kept to note the results.

The second class is trials of a new treatment when there is an existing treatment already. The question to be answered by the trial is whether the new treatment is an improvement on the old one. In such a case the normal trial would be between the existing and the new treatment. The use of placebos in such circumstances would be unethical, since it would amount to not treating a patient when in fact a treatment already exists, unless the condition is relatively minor (e.g. the common cold) and the patient has clearly consented to endure the discomfort of non-treatment if he happens to be given a placebo. If it is not possible to disguise the new treatment to make it appear like the existing one (which is the main advantage of placebos) then much larger groups will have to be used to avoid misleading results.

One particular ethical concern with therapeutic trials is that there is the potential for a blurring of the distinction between doctor and researcher. Doctors may often be involved in conducting these trials but the separate roles must be distinguished. We have already seen that among the presuppositions of the doctor-patient relationship are the assumption that the doctor will always act in the best interest of her patient and also that there will be truthfulness. This will be seriously undermined if the doctor involves her patient in a research project without his consent or abuses her position of relative power to pressurise a patient into agreeing. No one should have treatment forced on him against his wishes or without his consent, either explicit or given under pressure – even more so in the case of involvement in a research project.

Non-therapeutic trials raise less ethical questions because the research aspect is not complicated by the subject's need for medical treatment for his condition. The ethical considerations which should apply are those of any clinical trial, therapeutic or non-therapeutic. The subject must know as much as possible about the programme in order to give consent, including any known or suspected side-effects; the consent must be voluntary, and the subject's continuing autonomy must be preserved by ensuring he has the right to opt out at any time. It is clear therefore that consent is central to the ethical discussion of clinical trials.

The role of consent

In the earlier discussion of consent we saw that each person has the ability and must be allowed to make decisions about what is done to him in a medical situation. Each decision must be made by the patient in possession of all the facts (see chapter 2). The same applies in the area of research.

This can become an issue when trying to establish a suitable group. It is obviously important to eliminate as many variables as possible in the group to be tested, and groups like prisoners, members of the armed forces, school pupils, or long-stay patients in hospital or residents in a nursing home are very attractive groups since they share basic life-styles, diet, and so on. However, the principle of free consent to be an experimental subject still applies. Each person must give consent free of coercion, and it cannot be given on their behalf by a prison governor or matron etc. It is clearly wrong to coerce anyone into being an experimental subject.

The question of inducements is a further complication. It is doubtful if a general appeal to the public would produce a sufficient number of volunteers so it is common to offer payment. While it can be a useful source of income for many people, and people are entitled to be recompensed for any inconvenience involved, if those accepting it are desperate for money (e.g. down-and-outs) then a sense of coercion may be present even though unintended. So too with prisoners who may have volunteered freely, but the knowledge that better food and conditions are associated with the trial could form an irresistable inducement. Inducements or payments in themselves are not morally wrong, but in some situations may amount to a subtle form of coercion which would be morally very questionable.

The involvement of children: The need for free consent from each individual raises serious questions about the use of children for any such trial. This is a debate which occupies much ethical literature. The central issue is the limit to the right of parents (or guardians) to give consent on behalf of a minor. Again, in the discussion of consent earlier we saw that parental consent on behalf of a child is limited to what is in the best interest of the child (see page 19 above). They cannot consent to something which would endanger the life or health of their child. In the case of research it is argued that parents may only consent to their child being involved in therapeutic research, i.e. research which offers the hope of improvement in the condition of the child himself, and that parents can never consent to non-therapeutic research for their children.

One figure who argues in this way is the Protestant ethicist Paul Ramsey. He states that no-one 'can properly consent on another's behalf that this other become a subject of investigation primarily for the accumulation of scientific knowledge',[1] and sees children as the clearest case of this. Bernard Häring, the Roman Catholic writer, agrees. 'Besides informed parental or guardian consent, a second condition must be fulfilled, namely, that the medical investigation bear a definite relation to the treatment of the individual child and promise some advantage to him.'[2] There is widespread support for Ramsey and Häring on this strict line, but some disagree. Richard McCormick summarises an argument by Alan Porter from the *British Medical Journal* in favour of using children in non-therapeutic experiments when the risk is minimal. I quote it at length:

> He argues that there are grounds 'for believing that it may be permissible and reasonable to undertake minor precedures on children for experimental purposes with the permission of the parents.' The low risk/benefit ratio is the ultimate justification. Interestingly, Porter reports the reaction of colleagues and the public to a research protocol he had drawn up. He desired to study the siblings of children who had succumbed to 'cot death'. The research involved puncturing a vein (venipuncture). A pediatric authority told Porter that venipuncture was inadmissable under the Medical Research Council code. Astonished, Porter showed the protocol to the first ten colleagues he met. The instinctive reaction of nine out of ten was: 'Of course you may.' Similarly, a professional market researcher asked (for Porter) ten laymen about the procedure, and all responded that he could proceed. In other words, Porter argues that public opinion (and therefore, presumably, moral common sense) stands behind the low risk/benefit ratio approach to experimentation on children.[3]

The difference between Porter and Ramsey is the practical argument against the principled one. Not to pursue the sort of research Porter discusses would impede the progress of medical knowledge unnecessarily. However Ramsey would be unmoved by this argument – the principle involved is much too important. 'What is at stake here [in experiments on children] is the covenantal obligations of parents to children – the protection with which a child should be surrounded, and the meaning and duties of parenthood.'[4]

Moving even further from Ramsey and Häring's position is the *Declaration of Helsinki*, widely regarded as a basic document for guidelines on clinical research.[5] On non-therapeutic clinical research it states quite simply: 'Clinical research on a human being cannot be undertaken without his free consent after he has been informed; if he is legally incompetent, the consent of the legal guardian should be procured.'[6] In the case of children this would appear to stretch the limits of parental consent much further in the area of clinical research than is acceptable in other areas of medicine (e.g. the right to refuse a blood transfusion on behalf of a child).

And so the debate continues. One can see the logic and principles underlying the attitude of Ramsey and Häring, and yet understand Porter's appeal for tolerance of very minor procedures with very low risk but with the potential for immense benefit. The difficulty is that in moving away from the total ban on children in non-therapeutic trials one moves into an area of opinion and judgment, which is notoriously hard to control and prevent from inching forward. If one wants to move in the direction Porter wishes, then some sort of supervisory and regulatory control would appear to be essential.

Though this part of the discussion has centred on children in clinical research, it can be applied directly to all who are unable to consent for themselves – the mentally retarded person or the unconscious patient, for example.

Points for discussion or reflection

1. Should parents have the right to consent to their children being subjects in non-therapeutic trials where there is minimal risk?

2. How much information should be given to a patient who consents to being a subject in a therapeutic trial? Since the patient is ill, is there information which should not be disclosed?

3. Should doctors be forbidden to conduct clinical trials involving their own patients, in order to avoid a conflict between their role as doctor and their role as researcher?

4. It was stated that in the case of non-therapeutic trials the subject must have the right to opt out at any time. Does this mean that trials under anaesthetic can never be undertaken?

Notes:
1. P. Ramsey, *The Patient as Person* (Yale, 1970), p 20.
2. B. Häring, *Medical Ethics*, 3rd ed. (St. Paul, 1991), pp 200-201.
3. R. McCormick, *How Brave a New World?* (SCM, 1981) pp 57-8. The original article by Porter and others is in the *British Medical Journal*, 2 (1973), p 402.
4. Ramsey, op.cit. p 36.
5. *Declaration of Helsinki: Recommendations Guiding Doctors in Clinical Research*, a resolution adopted at the eighteenth World Medical Assembly in June 1964 by the World Medical Association.
6. ibid. Clause III 3a.

CHAPTER 9

Ethics and the Hospital: One Aspect

Some issues which arise in medical ethics are controversial, that is, there are sincerely held differences of opinion on their morality. Such include sterilisation, abortion, and some treatments for infertility such as IVF. These issues are first and foremost issues for the patient and for the medical staff concerned and we have already looked at the principles involved for these people in Chapter 2.

However a further question arises as to the way in which controversial issues ought to be handled in a hospital. Hospital authorities must decide whether facilities should be provided for such techniques and treatments, and if so, under what conditions and limitations. Sometimes a hospital may be governed by a particular ethos (e.g. a Roman Catholic hospital) which may either implicitly or explicitly forbid certain procedures. If so, what about the patient's right to disagree with the hospital ethos, and how are those patients' rights to be respected?

This issue is not one which arises only for hospitals. It is part of a much wider issue for society as a whole – how does society cater for those who disagree with the view of the majority on a significant issue? The rights of ethnic, religious, linguistic, and other minorities is an issue for most Western and democratic societies today. So I intend to look at one way in which the issue can be understood in society, before looking specifically at the issue for hospital authorities.

The social context

A very useful way to address this issue is to look at a well-known discussion in the history of social ethics – the Hart/Devlin debate. It arose in Britain in the 1960s, but the issues raised have much wider relevance, and it has surfaced in one form or other in most Western societies.

From time to time, most states have to face proposals for a change in the law relating to moral issues such as homosexuality, divorce, pornography, and so on. Those who argue for a liberalisation of the law usually argue that individuals should have the right to decide such issues for themselves, free from interference by the law; those opposed to such liberalisation often argue that the common good is paramount, and may have to take precedent over personal moral opinions. At the philosophical level, the debate is well represented by Lord Devlin on one hand, and by H. L. A. Hart on the other.

The argument against liberalising the law on many moral issues was put forward Lord Devlin in a book entitled *The Enforcement of Morals*.[1] He argued that an important responsibility of law is to protect society, and this includes its moral standards, since a society can be destroyed when there are no commonly accepted standards. The law therefore is justified in enforcing moral standards.

An alternative viewpoint was expressed by H. L. A. Hart in a book entitled *Law, Liberty, and Morality*,[2] where, while not denying what Devlin said about society, he argued that 'there must remain a realm of private morality which is, in brief and crude terms, not the law's business.'[3]

We have here two very different ways of understanding the role of law in areas of private morality. In effect, Devlin is arguing that the law is justified in interfering in what is often called private morality in order to uphold generally agreed moral standards and so protect society (i.e. to act for the common good). Hart argues the opposite. The state should not be involved in the area of private morality except to prevent a person doing harm to himself or another. The only role of law beyond that is to mark out the limits of reasonable choice.

Neither side is without its critics. How would Devlin establish what the generally accepted moral standards are? Presumably by finding out the opinions of the majority on a particular issue – perhaps by referendum. However this will create a minority who may find themselves bound against their judgment to the views of the majority. For example, a majority might find divorce unacceptable, but what of the minority who believe couples should have the right under certain circumstances to end their marriage and re-marry?

Hart's critics usually point to the difficulty in defining what private morality is. It is virtually impossible to outline any moral action which does not have an effect, no matter how indirect, on at least one other person. His defenders often respond by saying that if the major effect is on the individual, with an insignificant effect on the general public, then that action is private; otherwise it is public. But even this does not completely answer the criticism.

A refinement of Devlin's approach can be seen in those who argue that if something is wrong, then it is wrong not just for those who believe it is wrong, but it is also wrong even for those who believe it is right. For example, many who believe homosexual acts are wrong believe they are wrong even for those who do not believe they are wrong. In such a situation, they may argue that it is valid to try to seek a majority who agree with them and to use the law to 'enforce' moral behaviour on the minority.

Opponents of this approach would argue that, since it is a private matter between the two people concerned and so long as no one is harmed, then the law should not be involved at all. Anyway, it is argued, you cannot make people moral; conforming to the law is not the same as acting morally.

Versions of the Hart/Devlin debate can be seen to arise in various forms in countries worldwide as societies struggle to establish an appropriate response to a diversity of opinions on various moral issues that arise – often centring on subjects like divorce, homosexuality, abortion, or pornography.

Hospital policy
Depending on the way health services are organised within a

state, one may find different groups with responsibility for certain hospitals or clinics. This is most likely to arise when independent, voluntary or private institutions are incorporated into the health services, rather than in a state-controlled service. Such groups may be formally organised, like churches (Roman Catholic, Lutheran, Protestant) or groups related to churches such as religious orders, or religions (Jewish, Muslim), or more informal groups brought together for a particular purpose (e.g. family planning clinics), or simply a group of investors who build a hospital.

Such groupings will often have a viewpoint on particular moral questions which arise in medical practice, and because they control the hospital, they can control the availability of controversial treatments or procedures, either formally, by stating in a charter or foundation document that specific treatments will or will not be available; or more covertly, by ensuring that funding for certain treatments will or will not be available.

Any such body of people charged with the provision of health care in an area of the health service is entitled to have a viewpoint on controversial medical procedures and to have that expressed within the institution, either by permitting or forbidding the procedures. As such it is exercising as a corporate body the same right that any doctor has, not to be obliged to perform or assist at any treatment or procedure against her conscience. For example, a hospital under Roman Catholic management in a country where abortions are permitted, has the right to say that abortions will not be performed in that institution, just as a doctor has the right to refuse to perform or assist at an abortion if it is against her conscience.

However, to continue the analogy between the individual doctor and the hospital authorities, the doctor must be open with the patient as to the grounds for her refusal, and so too should the hospital authorities. It is very desirable therefore that policy on issues which might be controversial should be stated openly in a policy document or charter, rather than expressed in an underhand way by simply not making the facilities available.

The ethics committee

A more complex issue arises when morally controversial treatments are permitted within a hospital in certain circumstances, and debate often surrounds the way in which decisions about those treatments are managed. The Hart/Devlin discussion above now becomes relevant as a way of understanding differences of approach.

To take a common but sometimes morally sensitive procedure – sterilisation (either male vasectomy or female tubal ligation). In contexts where this procedure is morally sensitive it is sometimes the practice to issue guidelines (e.g. the patient must be over a certain age, have had some children, have partner's consent, etc) and further require that all such cases be referred to an ethics committee for approval. The committee usually comprises representatives of hospital management and staff, and sometimes of the wider community outside the hospital. The doctor interviews the patient and gathers the necessary information, which is then passed on to the committee (usually without disclosing the patient's identity), which then gives its decision.

If one sees the hospital as a microcosm of society as a whole, then what is happening is akin to the Devlin approach already mentioned. The hospital as a whole, through its ethics committee, is being asked to judge on the appropriateness of sterilisation in a particular case, and the individuals concerned, in this case the doctor and the patient, are bound by the committee's decision, irrespective of whether they agree with it or not.

An alternative approach sees the decision lying solely between the doctor and the patient. The doctor may be bound by guidelines laid down by the hospital authorities, but the authorities are not involved in individual decisions. The parallel with Hart's viewpoint should be obvious. The decision is a private one, and the only function of the hospital is to mark out the limits to that decision in accordance with its policy.

It is important to note that the difference between these two approaches is not the content of the guidelines nor the decisions of ethics committees – it is the existence or non-existence of the committee which is the issue. The fact that there is such a committee implies a certain understanding of the rights of an individual to make personal moral choices in the hospital context.[4]

The responsibility of the state: It is clear that where ethics committees exist they may have the effect of denying patients access to particular procedures or treatments which are legal and morally acceptable to the patient and are not contrary to sound medical opinion. Further, some institutions may legimately refuse to perform some medically sensitive procedures.

The net effect of all of this may be to limit the patient's access to treatment which he seeks and to restrict his right to decide what is in his best interest. The role of the state in respect of this must be to ensure the widest possible choice within the health service as a whole, provided such choice is within limits laid down by law, is reasonable to request, and accords with sound medical advice.

Other types of ethics committees: This discussion has centred on one particular type of ethics committee which has been controversial, but we must acknowledge that there are other types which are largely uncontroversial. Their role is usually to examine and report on the ethical implications of new forms of treatment or research, and to help those involved uncover the moral assumptions and consequences involved. Such bodies are obviously important as medicine and medical technology grows in complexity and provide an important service to the profession.

Points for discussion or reflection

1. Should all questions of private morality be questions solely for personal decision?

2. To what extent should decisions of a doctor and her patient on morally sensitive issues be constrained by an ethics committee or hospital policy?

3. Ought the state provide facilities for the full range of ethical opinion on medical issues? If there are to be limits on the state's obligations, how should they be decided?

Notes:
1. P. Devlin, *The Enforcement of Morals*, (OUP,1965)
2. H. L. A. Hart, *Law, Liberty, and Morality*, (OUP,1963)
3. ibid, pp 14-15.
4. Irish readers will recognise this as a central issue in the debate about the structure and management of the Adelaide Hospital at Tallaght, Dublin, during the 1980s and early 1990s.

CHAPTER 10

Allocation of Scarce Resources

Healthcare costs, as we all know, have risen consistently faster than inflation for many years now and are now so high that financial provision for them is becoming a serious issue in most societies. This is true whether we are dealing with a state funded system or one financed by private insurance and personal contributions, or a mixture of both. The reasons for the high costs are many but include the fact that as medicine achieves success in treating or eradicating more and more common illnesses, the emphasis has shifted to rarer and less easily treated illnesses. Also, the ability of medical technology to overcome many handicaps and alleviate suffering has led to a demand for the widespread availability of the treatment. All this has brought enormous benefits to the health and well-being of people and communities, but it has been accompanied by spiralling costs. To give a simple illustration: up to quite recently a person with a hip problem was given a (low cost) walking stick; today a (high cost) hip replacement is an option which brings a dramatic improvement in the person's quality of life.

Finance is the most common limitation on the availability of resources, but it isn't the only one. For many years access to kidney dialysis was limited because there simply weren't enough machines in existence. Today heart and other transplants are limited by the availability of willing and suitable donors.

So how do we decide priorities in such situations? How do we decide who should get treatment and who should not? Or, as the question is often very dramatically put, who should live when not all can live and yet not all need die?

Two famous cases

There are two cases which often form the basis for discussion of this issue in ethical literature. One is the case of a public committee set up in the Swedish Hospital in Seattle to select patients for a kidney machine; the other is the lifeboat example, which isn't a medical case at all, but analogies have been drawn between it and medical situations.

The Swedish Hospital committee:[1] In the late 1950s and early 1960s the Swedish Hospital in Seattle in the United States had to decide how it would control access to a kidney machine which could provide a totally effective way of saving the lives of very many people suffering with renal failure, and yet, because of cost, would not be available to everyone who could benefit from it.

A 'public committee' was set up – 'The Admissions and Policies Committee of the Seattle Artificial Kidney Center at Swedish Hospital' – to decide who should receive treatment. Medical advice suggested they reject children and anyone over forty-five automatically because of the poor prognosis for these categories at the time, and these weren't submitted to the committee. The membership of the committee remained anonymous, but was composed of medical and non-medical people, and was given the following information about each patient – age, sex, marital status, number of dependents, income, net worth, emotional stability (especially the patient's capacity to accept the treatment), education, occupation, past performance and future potential, and also the names of some referees for each patient.

One has only to put oneself for a moment in the position of the committee to realise how difficult its task was. How does one choose between a man with a young wife and three children, and one with an older wife with six children? – should the fact that the younger widow might have a greater opportunity to remarry be a factor? Does the fact that one has a substantial insurance policy and so his widow and children would be provided for influence the decision?

Paul Ramsey quotes a damning review of the work of the committee, 'presenting "a disturbing picture of the bourgeoise spar-

ing the bourgeoise" and concluding that "justice requires that
selection be made by a fairer method than the unbridled con-
sciences, the built-in biases and the fantasies of omnipotence of a
secret committee."'[2]

The lifeboat:[3] Suppose a group in a lifeboat determines that unless
some are sent overboard (to drown) then all will certainly die. Is
it acceptable to do so and how should one decide who is to
drown? Two legal cases surrounding actual cases are cited where
just such decisions were addressed – one American, the other
English. The American court accepted that a lottery among the
passengers was the only just way to decide who should die. The
English case rejected such a lottery as 'grotesque' and ruled that
all must wait and die or be rescued together. 'Who shall know
when masts and sails of rescue may emerge out of the fog?'[4]

Without discussing them in any depth, these two cases introduce the problems associated with making decisions about allocating limited resources.

How can we decide?

In practical terms there appear to be at least four options open to
us in the allocation of limited resources. They are: 1) Market
forces; 2) Desert; 3) Contribution to society; 4) A lottery.

1) Market forces: This is the simplest and probably the most common system of allocation, by which those who can afford expensive, life-saving treatment get it. It's very often part of a mixed
system where the state provides a certain level of health care for
all, for which the poorest at least don't have to pay. Those who
can afford it can buy more elaborate and expensive treatment in
the private sector, and for them the sky's the limit. The existence
of expensive private clinics in most Western countries represents
tacit acceptance of this system.

This is not the occasion to discuss in depth the question of
whether inequalities in wealth can be considered just. It can be
argued that because a person works harder, puts more effort
into his work, risks more, or contributes more to society, he/she
is entitled to higher renumeration and to the benefits that that

higher income brings, including, in this instance, better health care.

However, it can also be argued that health care and wealth cannot be associated in this way. Wealth is not based on need, and health care is. Those who most need health care are not obviously those who can best afford it. In fact the opposite may be the case – those living in poverty often need more health care than those who are wealthy.

2) *Desert:* Unlike market forces, there is no widespread acceptance of desert as a basis for distribution of scarce resources, but one occasionally hears modified versions of it, as for example when proposals are made that smokers should have lower priority in access to medical procedures if their condition is caused by smoking.

At the basis of a desert approach is a distinction between illnesses perceived to be random, and others where the lifestyle of the sufferer has contributed to the occurence of illness. Only those who deserve treatment should get it, it is argued; those who bring it on themselves don't deserve the same access to treatment, or at least should have a lower priority. Those who act in such a way as to bring illness on themselves ought not be allowed burden society with the cost of treatment.

Whatever plausibility such an approach might have in theory it doesn't work in practice. Gene Outka gives the following list of bidders for emergency care: '(1) a person with a heart attack who is seriously overweight; (2) a football hero who has suffered a concussion; (3) a man with lung cancer who has smoked cigarettes for forty years; (4) a sixty-year-old man who has always taken care of himself and is suddenly struck with leukemia; (5) a three-year-old girl who has swallowed poison left out carelessly by her parents; (6) a fourteen-year-old boy who has been beaten without provocation by a gang and suffers brain damage and recurrent attacks of uncontrollable terror; (7) a college student who has slashed his wrists (and not for the first time) from a psychological need for attention; (8) a woman raised in a ghetto who is found unconscious due to an overdose of heroin'.[5]

Consideration of any such list of real-life situations will show the impracticability of discriminating on the grounds of desert, and this will become even more complex the more we probe into the patient's background. We must also be aware that some people are simply unwilling to face facts and accept warnings about their health, often for deep psychological reasons.

3) Contribution to society: This approach places emphasis on concepts such as the public interest, the common good, the welfare of the community, or the greatest good for the greatest number of people. In so far as it considered criteria such as age, dependents, occupation, and so on, the Swedish Hospital Committee may be seen to have taken this sort of approach.

There are two ways this can be approached – by looking at particular groups and their value to society (e.g. mothers of young children, wage earners, highly skilled professions, etc) and giving them priority; or assessing the value of each individual and organising a hierarchy of 'valuable people' in this way, which is what the Swedish Hospital Committee attempted.

As we saw earlier, the committee failed to produce any widely acceptable criteria for assessing the relative value of groups or individuals. Many would say it is ethically unacceptable even to attempt it. The basis of our response to another person in need is the fact that he is in need, not some value he may contribute if he is saved. To take it out of the medical field, we feel a responsibility to help those affected by famine or drought in the third world, not because they have the potential to make an important contribution to global society, but because they are there, they are human, and they are in need. That's sufficient. It would be 'inhuman' to attempt to assess their value and worth before offering aid.

4) Lottery: It is out of a sense of a common humanity and the basic equality of all human beings that most favour a lottery as the only just way to distribute limited resources. This is the approach favoured by Paul Ramsey, for example, who says 'life is a value incommensurate with all others, and so is not negotiable by bartering one man's life against another's'. 'The equal right of every human being to live, and not relative personal or social worth, should be the ruling principle. When not all can be saved and all need not die, this ruling principle can be applied only or best by a random choice among equals.'[6] Here the lifeboat case is relevant, and Ramsey and others are favouring the American court's decision that, in the end, a lottery is the only way to decide.

This lottery can operate in two ways – either a simple lottery where names are literally put in a hat, or on the basis of 'first come, first served', which is a form of ongoing lottery. Many will find the use of a hat as too trivial when human life is concerned. The queue is something we are much more used to and so find acceptable, though some will be surprised to hear it described as a lottery.

I'm inclined to follow Ramsey in his support for the lottery. It is rooted in the basic equality of all human beings and in the equal right to life we all possess. I would, however, impose two conditions before the lottery is applied:

(a) Every effort must be made to eliminate the need for such lotteries. There is some merit in the English court's judgment in the lifeboat case which saw a lottery as grotesque, and while few would support its conclusions by arguing that therefore we must never choose and so save no one's life, a more sensible conclusion is that such choices should be avoided if possible. There is something demeaning to human worth to tell a person 'we know how to save your life or alleviate your suffering but can't afford it'. Choices about allocating limited resources may be unavoidable, but are not desirable. So, in my opinion, priority should be given to providing sufficient resources to avoid scarcity in one area (and so remove the need for a choice), before introducing a limited facility in another area; for example, placing emphasis on providing kidney machines for all who need them, before introducing heart transplants for some, and so adding to the occurrence of scarcity.

(b) Before introducing a person to the lottery (or queue) or beginning treatment, there should be a probability of 'lasting success', to use Häring's phrase.[7] This is especially important with a queue, where it may happen that by the time a person reaches the head of the queue his medical condition may have deteriorated to such an extent that the treatment may not offer such a probability.

Points for discussion or reflection

1. Did the Swedish Hospital public committee fail because of the criteria it used, or was the attempt wrong in principle?

2. Construct full ethical defences for *both* court decisions in the 'lifeboat' cases. Which aspects are decisive for you?

3. Do you agree that a lottery is the only way to distribute scarce resources? What are its disadvantages?

Notes:
1. The most accessible account is in P. Ramsey, *The Patient as Person* (Yale, 1970), pp 242ff.
2. ibid, p 248.
3. Again Ramsey provides the most accessible account, p 253.
4. ibid, p 253, n 4.
5. G. Outka, 'Social Justice and Equal Access to Health Care', in T.A. Shannon (ed), *Bioethics* (Paulist, 1981), p 483.
6. P. Ramsey, op. cit., p 256.
7. B. Häring, *Medical Ethics*, 3rd ed (St Paul, 1991), p 192.

CHAPTER 11

AIDS

Few issues have had such a profound effect on medical and ethical thinking this century as the discovery of AIDS. The emergence of a completely new terminal and as yet incurable illness mainly affecting young adults has made huge demands in the area of research and medical and hospice care, and consequent demands for substantial resources. Fears in the wider community about infection raised many questions about how this care was to be delivered, and also how its spread might be curtailed.

The discovery of AIDS has been the occasion of an outpouring of statements and discussions, often very profound, about the nature of health and illness, the questioning of lifestyles, and the modification of behaviour. It has also seen an excessive amount of pious and platitudinous moralising which often says more about the speaker than about the subject under discussion.

The Christian churches too have been forced to reassess their position on many issues in the light of AIDS. They have been pushed to think again their attitudes to relationships, and how to express that tradition in the light of new circumstances. The traditional Christian commitment to healthcare and pioneering work in hospice care has been a major resource, but this contribution has sometimes been damaged by confused thinking on some moral questions associated with AIDS.

The chief features of AIDS and the main ways in which it is spread are too well known to be repeated here, so in this chapter I will concentrate on two aspects of this whole discussion – (a) the Christian response, and some personal comments on it; and (b) specific ethical issues surrounding AIDS.

(a) The Christian response

There is a widespread perception that much of the initial Christian reaction to the discovery of AIDS was couched in 'wrath of God' language. Some of this was quite overt, especially among fringe fundamentalist groups who saw the disease as a vindication of Christian denouncements of immoral behaviour and an expression of the wrath of God on certain segments of society.

However this was not the response of the main churches, whose statements, especially in the early stages, often followed a similar pattern: an expression of genuine compassion, a call for adequate medical and research resources to be made available, and then there usually followed a re-affirmation of traditional Christian attitudes to sexual relationships and drug abuse and a warning that only by accepting Christian standards in these areas could the disease be avoided. This latter section is certainly not 'wrath of God' language, but there is a strong undercurrent of 'we warned you', 'we were right all along' in this sort of response. It is implicitly saying 'something bad will happen you unless you follow Christian standards. AIDS is the consequence of not following the Christian way'. This language of inevitable judgment can be seen as akin to, but much gentler than, wrath of God language.

This deserves to be explored much further. In hindsight, the initial reaction is not very surprising when one thinks of some of the main ways in which HIV and AIDS is transmitted one to another – through drug abuse, or promiscuous heterosexual or homosexual sexual activity – activities which Christians have condemned unequivocally for many years. In particular in the area of attitudes to sexual activity, Christians have frequently been accused of not moving with the times, of failing to face the reality of the current situation especially since the widespread availibility of reliable contraception. One can understand, even if one does not condone, a mild sense of self-satisfaction if it has now been discovered that promiscuity as well as drug abuse is 'very bad for your health'. One can almost hear the chant of 'I told you so' falling from the lips of some church people bruised and battered from the struggle to maintain their so called 'out-of-date sexual morality'.

In reply it must be pointed out that it is not just promiscuous sexual activity and drug abuse that put people at risk. People receiving blood transfusions and other blood products (especially haemophiliacs) were at serious risk until adequate blood screening techniques were introduced, and babies born to mothers with HIV infection have also been found to be infected. Frequently these latter cases were referred to as 'innocent victims', leaving unstated the notion that the other sufferers were 'guilty victims'. The question must then be asked – what are they guilty of, that they deserve AIDS?

The 'wrath of God' theory was very well answered in a much quoted sermon by Richard Holloway, the Anglican Bishop of Edinburgh, in 1986. Part of it is worth quoting at length:

> To argue that AIDS is God's punishment on homosexuals seems to me to be morally repugnant and illogical. Morally repugnant, because it creates a picture of God as an enraged terrorist who fashions and throws bombs at his enemies, no matter who gets injured. But it is also illogical, because it is inconsistent. ... It differentiates between male and female homosexuals, and seems to put the God who inspires scientific research against the God who dreams up new diseases in his great laboratory in the sky. But if it is argued that God does reward wickedness so specifically, why is he taking so long to lob something at rapists or child abusers, groups that are infinitely more malign in their effects than most gay men? No, the 'wrath of God' theory of AIDS discloses more about the attitudes of those who hold it than it does about the nature of God.[1]

The question of judgment deserves further consideration. In Christian thinking all societies and individuals stand under judgment; it is part of the understanding of the Fall that disorder is introduced into the world because of mankind's failure to live up to God's law.

This judgment is seen in many areas – in the failure of relationships, in the divide between haves and have-nots, in the existence of famine or nuclear disasters or other examples of the human abuse of nature. So also in health. Many diseases would not exist were it not for our failure to respect the divine ordering of creation, e.g. extreme stress or heart disease caused by lifestyle, some cancers caused by smoking or the use of asbestos. Such areas of suffering are not caused or sent by God, but it seems they follow from a failure, whether deliberate or unwitting, to live according to God's law.

Also, if we believe in any sense of natural law, it should not surprise us that what the Christian tradition commends on moral grounds should coincide with what health experts commend on medical grounds. However we cannot argue for or defend a moral position on the grounds that it is a health risk.

Christian attitudes to AIDS must be grounded in the virtues of care, compassion, freedom and justice, and must be careful to avoid presenting a moral iron fist in the soft glove of compassion and concern. Christians do have important values to share with society, particularly in the area of sexual morality and behaviour, especially their belief in the virtues of chastity and fidelity as some of the means whereby the highest degree of personal integrity and expression of love can be achieved. These values commend themselves on their own merit; they do not need the fear of a life-threatening disease to give them validity.

(b) Specific ethical issues

Ethical issues surrounding diagnosis: Since the period between infection and signs of illness can be several years, the test to establish whether one is infected or not is very important both for the individual who has the test and also for his/her recent sexual partners. Normally the individual who is tested is healthy at the time and, given the current state of knowledge and research, the news of a positive result is effectively telling a healthy person he has a terminal illness. It may also involve tracing and informing recent sexual partners and encouraging them to have the test. Family, friends, and colleagues may react differently to the information, and the person may be shunned by some or faced with irrational prejudice. In some cases it may involve disclosing for the first time to family or colleagues that one is gay or has been using drugs – news which may not be well received.

For all these reasons there is a moral responsibility on those performing the test to counsel the subject on all these issues so that he/she is prepared for all this should the test be positive.

Undergoing a test is not always done voluntarily – a test may be compulsory or made a condition for something the subject wishes to have. Compulsory mass screening of whole nations or of substantial groups within society was sometimes proposed in the early days of AIDS, but is probably totally impractical, since it would involve a huge commitment of medical workers and laboratory technicians for comparatively little benefit.

A more common form of mass screening is the routine testing for AIDS of blood samples sent to a laboratory for other reasons. The purpose is usually to establish the statistical occurrence of the condition in a given area so that future planning of resources can be made. One must be very careful about this. When one gives a blood sample there is either implicit or explicit consent by the patient. For example I may visit my GP because of an illness and she may suggest a blood test to help establish the cause. Unless AIDS is one of a number of suspected causes and this has been explained to me, the GP has no right to have the blood tested for AIDS without my consent. In effect to do this would be to force a test on me without my consent, which we have already seen would be unethical.[2]

On the other hand, one can see the advantages from a health authority's point of view of having statistical information about the occurrence of AIDS, information which would be readily available from blood samples already in the laboratory. It would, in my opinion, be acceptable for a health authority to routinely or randomly test blood samples for AIDS, provided this is done in such a way that a positive result could not be traced back to an individual patient. It would still produce the statistical information required. Some people may find this odd – why not tell the patient? Surely some would appreciate being told, even if it was bad news? However remember the principle of what is going on – the test was not sought by the patient or his GP. On what basis would the health authority be authorised to disclose the result to the patient? Yet the authority cannot hold information about a person which it has not disclosed to that person.[3]

In reply it may be argued that AIDS is an infectious disease which is life-threatening and so the normal rights about information and confidentiality do not apply.[4] However AIDS is not a threat to the general public; in fact it is only a threat to people who come into intimate contact with blood, semen or other body fluid of a person with the condition. It is not unreasonable to expect such people to take precautions against possible infection.

It is sometimes argued that the medical profession, because its members may come into contact with blood from their patients, has a right to know whether a patient is infected or not, and so has the right to test a patient without his consent in order to protect itself from infection. In fact the British Medical Association passed a resolution to this effect in 1987. However that decision was subsequently reversed following legal opinion. No one has the right to test a patient without his consent.

A not dissimilar situation arose for insurance companies. Obviously AIDS infection hugely affects life projections which are central to life assurance and pension calculations. Yet some clients might be put off or offended by being asked to agree to be tested. It was suggested that a test could be part of the general medical examination which is common with such insurance, but because of sensitivity to the test, it should not be disclosed to the client that this was being done and the result only made known to the company. Again this was rejected as unethical. Consent must be obtained for any test, and information from such a test should not be witheld from the client.

Consequences of a positive test: In normal situations when one has a positive result from a test for any condition, the results of that test remain confidential to the subject and his medical advisor. The only exception to this is when the condition may seriously threaten the life of a member of the general public.[5]

AIDS does not put the general public at risk, but it does put the subject's sexual partners at risk. It is already widely accepted that in the case of other sexually-transmitted diseases the responsibility for telling one's partner lies with the subject. Is this also the case with AIDS?

This is a very controversial issue. Some argue that confidentiality demands that the onus lies solely with the subject who is infected; others, that because the disease is life-threatening, a doctor is justified in telling the partner. In my opinion, the onus lies with the subject to disclose the results of the test to his partner. However if he obviously refuses to tell him/her and has been given ample opportunity to do so, then I believe a doctor may break confidentiality by telling the partner if it is practical to do so, on the grounds that it is a genuinely life-threatening condition, and the subject has no right to threaten the life of another person unnecessarily. However, I emphasise that this is my opinion, and it is not clear whether a court, for example, would support this.

Another consequence of a positive test centres on the question of abortion. When a woman becomes pregnant her immune system is supressed in the early stages of pregnancy. If she is HIV positive then pregnancy may substantially increase the chances of developing or at least advancing full AIDS. It has been argued that in such a situation pregnancy is life-threatening for the mother and so a termination of the pregnancy is justified. The morality of such an action then becomes part of the wider discussion of abortion (see chapter 5).

If a pregnant woman is HIV positive or has AIDS there is a very strong likehood that the baby will go on to develop AIDS. It is sometimes argued that this is akin to being born with such serious handicap that the baby won't survive, and so a termination is acceptable.[6] However there is some evidence that the baby may not go on to develop AIDS, and if this is the case it's hard to see how this argument can be sustained.

Allocation of resources: The various treatments so far available for AIDS are expensive. Given the rapid spread of the disease, it is likely in the future that its treatment will make huge demands on the financial and professional resources of health authorities. In deciding priorities in the allocation of budgets, it is possible that some of the lifestyles associated with the spread of AIDS may give rise to perhaps unstated prejudices against the allocation of adequate resources for AIDS prevention and treatment. The notion that some are 'guilty' has already been discussed and dismissed, but it is possible that it may surface in decisions about resource allocation.

AIDS is a disease like any other – more tragic than most since it mainly affects young people and at present is incurable. It is entitled to the same consideration by the same criteria in resource allocation as any other illness or condition. There is always the possibility that a subtle form of prejudice could be expressed against AIDS sufferers. Society as a whole must be extra vigilant against such prejudice.

Points for discussion or reflection

1. Outline what, in your opinion, would be an appropriate Christian response to AIDS.

2. What special questions does AIDS raise for the normal rule of confidentiality between doctor and patient?

3. Are there certain careers or professions which a person should resign if he or she is found to be HIV positive (e.g. surgeon, dentist, chef, waiter, first-aid volunteer)?

Notes:
1. R. Holloway, 'Some Pastoral and Ethical Implications of AIDS' (1986).
2. See p 16.
3. See pp 20.
4. See pp 23.
5. ibid.
6. see for example p 58.

Suggested further reading

General:

A. S. Duncan, G. R. Dunstan and R. B. Welbourn (eds), *A New Dictionary of Medical Ethics* (London: DLT, 1981, Rev ed).

B. Häring, *Medical Ethics* (Slough: St Paul, 1991, 3rd ed).

M. Lockwood (ed), *Moral Dilemmas in Modern Medicine* (Oxford, OUP, 1985).

R. McCormick, *How Brave a New World?* (London, SCM, 1981).

J. Mahoney, *Bioethics and Belief* (London: Sheed & Ward, 1984).

W. T. Reich, *Encyclopedia of Bioethics,* 2 vols, (London: Collier Macmillan, 1983, Rev ed).

P. Ramsey, *The Patient as Person* (Yale University Press, 1970).

T. A. Shannon (ed), *Bioethics* (New York, Paulist Press, 1993, 4th ed). Previous editions contain different selections of articles and should also be consulted.

Specific issues:

R. F. Gardner, *Abortion – The Personal Dilemma* (London, Paternoster Press, 1972).

D. J. Horan and D. Mall (eds), *Death, Dying and Euthanasia* (Marytland, 1980).

M. Reidy (ed), *Ethical Issues in Reproductive Medicine* (Dublin, Gill and Macmillan, 1982).

S. Sontag, *AIDS and its Metaphors* (Harmondsworth, Penguin Books, 1990).